D0402879

How We Do Harm

HOW WE DO HARM

A Doctor Breaks Ranks
About Being Sick in America

Otis Webb Brawley, M.D.,
with Paul Goldberg

St. Martin's Press New York

HOW WE DO HARM. Copyright © 2011 by Otis Webb Brawley, M.D., with Paul Goldberg. All rights reserved. Printed in the United States of America. For information, address St. Martin's Press, 175 Fifth Avenue, New York, N.Y. 10010.

www.stmartins.com

ISBN 978-0-312-67297-3

First Edition: January 2012

10   9   8   7   6   5   4   3   2   1

Contents

Part III.   More Is Better

Part IV.   Evidence-Based Medicine

Lord, teach me to be generous.

Teach me to serve you as you deserve;

to give and not to count the cost,

to fight and not to heed the wounds,

to toil and not to seek for rest,

to labor and not to ask for reward,

save that of knowing that I do your will.

—"Prayer for Generosity,"
ST. IGNATIUS OF LOYOLA

How We Do Harm

PART I

Three from the Gradys

Chapter 1

Chief Complaint

SHE WALKS THROUGH the emergency room doors sometime in the early morning. In a plastic bag, she carries an object wrapped in a moist towel.

She is not bleeding. She is not in shock. Her vital signs are okay. There is no reason to think that she will collapse on the spot. Since she is not truly an emergency patient, she is triaged to the back of the line, and other folks, those in immediate distress, get in for treatment ahead of her. She waits on a gurney in a cavernous, green hallway.

The "chief complaint" on her chart at Grady Memorial Hospital, in downtown Atlanta, might have set off a wave of nausea at a hospital in a white suburb or almost any place in the civilized world. It reads, "My breast has fallen off. Can you reattach it?"

She waits for at least four hours—likely, five or six. The triage nurse doesn't seek to determine the whereabouts of the breast.

Obviously, the breast is in the bag.

I am making rounds on the tenth floor when I get a page from Tammie Quest in the Emergency Department.

At Grady, we take care of patients who can't pay, patients no one wants. They come to us with their bleeding wounds, their run-amok diabetes, their end-stage tumors, their drama. You deal with this wreckage for a while and you develop a coping mechanism. You detach. That's why many doctors, nurses, and social workers here come off as if they have departed for a less turbulent planet.

3

Tammie is not like that. She emotes, and I like having her as the queen of ER—an experienced black woman who gives a shit. When Dr. Quest pages me, I know it isn't because she needs a social interaction. It has to be something serious.

"We are wanted in the ER," I tell my team.

The cancer team today consists of a fellow, a resident, two medical students, and yours truly, in a flowing white coat, as the attending physician. I lead the way down the hall. Having grown up Catholic, I can't help thinking of the med students and young doctors as altar boys following a priest.

I am a medical oncologist, the kind of doctor who gives chemotherapy. My other interests are epidemiology and biostatistics. I am someone you might ask whether a drug works, whether you should get a cancer screening test, and whether a white man's cancer differs from a black man's cancer. You can also ask me if we are winning the "war" on the cluster of diseases we call cancer. As chief medical officer of the American Cancer Society—a position I have held since 2007—I often end up quoted in the newspapers, and I am on television a lot. In addition to my academic, journalistic, and public-policy roles, I have been taking care of cancer patients at Grady for nearly a decade, first as the founding director of the cancer center, and now as chief doctor at the ACS.

My retinue behind me, I keep up a fast pace, this side of a jog. Bill Bernstein, the fellow, is the most senior of the group. Bill is a Newton, Massachusetts, suburbanite, still boyish. He is having trouble adjusting to the South, to Atlanta, to its inner city. He is trying, but it's hard to miss that black people and poor people perplex him. Contact with so much despair makes him awkward. But he has a good heart, a surfeit of common sense—and he is smart. Whatever we teach him at Grady will make him a better doctor wherever he ends up.

Grady suffers from what the administration here calls a "vertical transportation problem." Our elevators are slow at best, broken at worst. We head for the stairs, rushing down to the first floor, then through long, green hallways into the ER.

Grady is a monument to racism. Racism is built into it, as is poverty, as is despair. Shaped like a capital letter *H,* Grady is essentially two hospitals with a hallway—a crossover—in the middle to keep things separate but equal for sixteen stories.

In the 1950s and '60s, white patients were wheeled into the front section, which faces the city. Blacks went to the back of the *H*. This structure—built in 1953—was actually an improvement over the previous incarnation. The Big H—the current Grady—replaced two separate buildings—the whites got a brick building, the blacks a run-down wood-frame structure. Older Atlantans continue to refer to the place in a chilling plural, the Gradys.

You end up at Grady for four main reasons. It could happen because you have no insurance and are denied care at a private hospital, or because you are unconscious when you arrive by ambulance. When your lights are out, you are in no position to ask to be taken to a cleaner, better-lit, suburban palace of medicine. A third, small contingent are older black folks with insurance, who could go anywhere but have retained a dim memory of Grady as the only Atlanta hospital that accepted us. The fourth category, injured cops and firemen, know that we see a lot of shock and trauma and are good at it. We are their ER of choice.

Today, our 950-bed behemoth stands for another form of segregation: poor versus rich, separate but with no pretense of equality. Grady is Atlanta's safety-net hospital. It is also the largest hospital in the United States.

The ER, arguably the principal entry point to Grady, was built in the center of the hospital, filling in some of the *H* on the first floor. To build it, Grady administrators got some federal funds in time for the 1996 Summer Olympics. This fueled financial machinations, which led to criminal charges, which led to prison terms. (In retrospect, the bulk of the money was put to good use. Many of the victims of the Olympic Park bombing came through our ER.)

The hallways here are incredibly crowded, even by the standards of inner-city hospitals. Patients are triaged into three color-coded lines—surgery, internal medicine, obstetrics—and placed on gurneys two-deep, leaving almost no room for staff to squeeze through.

You might see a homeless woman drifting in and out of consciousness next to a Georgia Tech student bloodied from being pistol-whipped in an armed robbery, next to a fifty-seven-year-old suburban secretary terrified by a sudden loss of vision, next to a twenty-eight-year-old hooker writhing in pain that shoots up from her lower abdomen, next to a conventioneer who blacked out briefly in a cylindrical tower of a downtown hotel, next to a fourteen-year-old slum dweller who struggles for breath as his asthma attack subsides.

When I first arrived in Atlanta and all of this was new to me, I took my wife, Yolanda, through the Grady ER on a Friday night.

"Oh, the humanity," she said.

Yolanda, a lawyer with the U.S. Securities and Exchange Commission, feels happier above the Mason-Dixon Line.

TAMMIE Quest—I use her real name—is cute, has a broad, infectious smile, and comes from privilege. She grew up in Southern California and frequently refers to herself as a "black Valley girl."

Though she identifies with the West Coast, a lot of Atlanta has rubbed off on her in the Grady ER.

No two ERs are alike. Ours tells the story of Atlanta more clearly, more poignantly than its skyline. Patients everywhere are scared of their wounds or diseases that rage inside them. Here, in the middle of this big, hot, loud, violent city, they have an added fear: they are terrified of each other, often with good cause.

Elsewhere, patients might trust us doctors, admire us, even bow to our robes, our honorifics, and the all-caps abbreviations that follow our names. Here, not so much.

A place called Tuskegee is about two hours away from here. It's where government doctors staged a medical experiment in the thirties: they watched black men die of syphilis, withholding treatment even after effective drugs were invented.

Tuskegee is not an abstraction in these parts. It's a physical place, as palpable as a big, deep wound, and eighty-plus years don't mean a thing. Tuskegee is a huge, flashing CAUTION sign in the consciousness of Southern black folks. It explains why they don't trust doctors much and why good docs such as Tammie have to fight so hard to earn their elementary trust.

Like me, Tammie is a member of the medical-school faculty at Emory University, and, like me, she has several academic interests. One of these interests is end-of-life care for cancer patients: controlling the symptoms when someone with advanced cancer shows up in your ER.

Seeing us approach, she walks toward us and hands me a wooden clipboard with the Grady forms. I look at her face, gauging the mixture of sadness, moral outrage, and fatigue.

She says something like "This patient *needs* someone who cares," and disappears.

I glance at the chief complaint.

"Holy shit," I say to Bill Bernstein and, more so, to myself.

I introduce myself to a trim, middle-aged, black woman, not unattractive, wearing a blue examination gown conspicuously stamped GRADY. (At Grady, things such as gowns, infusion pumps, and money tend to vanish.)

From the moment Tammie paged me, I knew that the situation had to be more than a run-of-the-mill emergency. This patient clearly is not about to die on the examination table. She doesn't need emergency treatment. Before anything, she needs somebody to talk to. She needs attention, both medical and human.

The patient, Edna Riggs, is fifty-three. She works for the phone company and lives on the southeast side of Atlanta.

Sitting on an exam table, she looks placid. When she extends her hand, it feels limp. She makes fleeting eye contact. This is depression, maybe. Shame does the same thing, as does a sense of doom. *Fatalism* is the word doctors have repurposed to describe this last form of alienation.

In medicine, we speak a language of our own, and Edna's physical problem has a name in doctorese: automastectomy. It's a fancy way of saying that the patient's breast has fallen off by itself.

An automastectomy can occur when a tumor grows so big and so deep that it cuts off the blood supply from the chest to the breast. Denied oxygen, breast tissue dies and the breast starts to detach from the chest wall. At places such as Grady, automastectomies are seen a couple of times a year, often enough to be taken in stride.

This case is different from others I have seen only because Edna Riggs has wrapped her detached breast in a moist, light-blue towel and brought it with her for reattachment. I can't help wondering why the towel is moist. Some deliberateness has gone into the breast's care. I cringe at the thought that Edna has kept that package next to her on the gurney in the ER for hours.

In the exam gown, Edna's chest looks surprisingly normal. I ask how long she has had a "breast problem."

She first felt something in her breast when her son was in second grade, she replies. It has grown over the years. She speaks correct English, not the language of the streets. She sounds like someone who has had schooling, a person who reads. Her hair is clean and combed, she is dressed neatly.

What grade is her son in now?

Eleventh.

I don't react, not visibly. She has known she had a problem for nine years—why did she do nothing?

I ask Edna's permission to examine her. She nods. I ask her to lie down, my entourage gathering around.

I help her remove her right arm from the gown, trying to respect her modesty and preserve as much dignity as possible. I undrape the right breast, or the place where the right breast had been. The chest wall is now rugged. I see yellowish, fibrous tissue and dry blood. There is the unforgettable smell of anaerobic bacteria. The wound is infected.

I reach for examination gloves. I palpate her chest wall and feel under her armpit, looking for evidence of enlarged nodes. After examining the breast wall, I look in the towel. Her amputated breast could fit on her chest as if it were a puzzle piece.

I am not looking forward to Edna's repeating her request to reattach the breast. If she asks directly, I will have to say that this is not possible and explain why not. My preference is to move slowly, to let her adjust, to make her comfortable with me, with receiving medical care for her condition. I fear that she will get up, leave, and never return. Fortunately, Edna doesn't repeat her request. Perhaps the magnitude of the problem confronting her is starting to sink in.

Edna's breast cancer has been growing for at least nine years. It's unheard-of that cancer such as this would be anything but metastatic.

The disease has to have disseminated to her bones, lungs, brain, liver. I feel a wave of frustration and anger.

Another day at Grady Memorial Hospital. Here I sit, talking with a patient whom we would probably have cured nine years earlier, and today I will have to tell her that she has a terminal disease.

The rest is logistics. I arrange for the pathology and radiology to get confirmation. We always get pathologic confirmation of cancer, even when we are almost certain that it is cancer. An old medical saying goes: "When you hear hoofbeats, think horses, not zebras." This saying has an important corollary: "You don't want to be bit on the ass by a zebra." There is a remote possibility that Edna's automastectomy was caused by leprosy or some unusual infectious disease. It's cheap and easy to get verification that it's cancer.

I ask Bill Bernstein to talk with Edna, to take a full history, to perform a full examination. The objective is to rule out neurologic problems from spread of the disease to the brain or spine, to look for other evidence of problems caused by the disease.

If you take me aside and ask why I'm withdrawing from the scene, I will say that I am trying to awaken Bill's compassion. But it is something else as well, something about me. I am afraid of growing callous. I acknowledge this readily, as a means of staving it off. I am trying to avoid accepting the unnecessary loss of yet another life. In the case of Edna Riggs, the abstract, scholarly term *health disparities* acquires a very real smell of a rotting breast.

I take my leave and, with the resident, start arranging tests to confirm the diagnosis and get Edna ready for treatment. We will fight, even though we are going to lose. Metastatic breast cancer always wins. We have drugs to decrease pain and even make most people live longer, but we can beat breast cancer only when it's caught early.

WE admit Edna Riggs into the hospital, to get the tests done and to start antibiotic treatment of the infected wound. We could have done the workup without admitting her, but I fear that she will leave the system as abruptly as she entered. Psychological and emotional support are legitimate reasons for admittance, though most insurance companies and Medicaid would disagree.

As she starts to trust me, Edna tells me how frightened she was when she found a lump in her breast. Right away, she knew it was breast cancer, and in her experience, everyone who got breast cancer died quickly, painfully. Insurance problems kept her away from the doctor, as did the fear of dying. She knew she would die after going to the doctor. Several of her friends had.

Early on, Edna had some insurance, which didn't do her any good. Her employer wouldn't let her take just two or three hours of sick leave to go to the doctor. If she needed to take sick leave, she had to take it in increments of one day. This guaranteed that an employee would exhaust all the leave quickly. If Edna had been fired for taking time off after exhausting her sick leave, her three kids, too, would have lost support and insurance.

Acknowledging the physical problem and facing the consequences became increasingly difficult. Edna tells me that she feared the disease, but she also feared the system. Would the doctors scold her? Would they experiment on her? Would they give her drugs that caused nausea, vomiting, hair loss? Would the hospital kill her?

Edna's decision to stay out of the medical system was about fear: fear of breast cancer, fear of the medical profession, fear of losing the roof over her kids' heads. Fear intensified after her employer started to require copayments from workers who wanted to be insured. This extra $3,000 a year made health insurance too expensive to keep.

Payment for medical services and sick-leave policies determine the quality of care we receive. Several years ago, my research team at the American Cancer Society published data showing that people diagnosed with cancer who had no insurance or were insured through Medicaid were 1.6 times more likely to die in five years as those with private insurance.

In breast cancer, patients with private insurance were more likely to be diagnosed with Stage I breast cancer than those who had no insurance or were receiving Medicaid.

In colon cancer, too, the chances of catching the disease at an earlier, treatable stage were lower in the uninsured and Medicaid populations.

Even when the disease was found early, an uninsured patient did worse than one with insurance. For example, an insured patient with Stage II colon cancer had better odds of being alive five years after diagnosis than an uninsured patient with what should be highly curable Stage I cancer.

Another study focused on emergency surgery to treat bowel perforation, peritonitis, or obstruction in colon-cancer patients under age sixty-five. This surgical emergency was 2.6 times more frequent in uninsured patients than in those with private insurance. Among patients receiving Medicaid, the odds of needing this surgery was 2.1 times higher than in those with private coverage.

ACS epidemiologists estimate that the lack of insurance annually costs eight thousand Americans their lives due to inability to receive cancer treatment. Even controlling cancer pain is no small challenge if you are poor. Uninsured patients cannot afford pain medicines. The social programs that give them medication heavily ration pain meds.

Even if you have insurance that will pay for your treatment, you may still not be able to afford to receive it.

I have seen poor breast-cancer patients choose mastectomy (surgical removal of the entire breast) over a lumpectomy (removal of the tumor) because of employer sick-leave policies. A woman who chooses a lumpectomy must also receive radiation, which has to be given daily, Monday through Friday, for six to eight weeks. The treatment requires fifteen minutes in the clinic, but it's done only during business hours. Unfortunately, this less disfiguring treatment is hardly an option for a woman who knows that longer postoperative treatment will cause her to lose her job.

Most states have laws that require doctors to tell the patients that they have a choice of full removal of the breast or removal of the cancerous lump with follow-up radiation. I do better than that. I tell my patients that I believe that lumpectomy with radiation is a better option, as it is less deforming and likely to lead to less long-term swelling.

PATIENTS most likely to have the worst outcomes are defined in a couple of ways. Poverty is the biggest driver, followed by race. (Race is complicated. For now, let's think of it as just another snippet of data collected from cancer patients, and delve into its significance later.)

Much of the problem is that poor people don't get care that would be likely to help them. The reasons for this are complex. Perhaps they can't

get care, or don't know where care is available, or they haven't been offered insurance or steady access to care by their jobs or social services.

Here is the problem: Poor Americans consume too little health care, especially preventive health care. Other Americans—often rich Americans—
consume too much health care, often unwisely, and sometimes to their
detriment. The American health-care system combines famine with gluttony.

We could improve dismal health outcomes on both ends of the socioeconomic spectrum if we were simply faithful to science, if we provided
and practiced care that we know to be effective.

EARLY on, Edna ignored her tumor. She accomplished this easily during
her busy days, but not when she was alone at night.

The disease progressed relentlessly. The lump grew. Then the tumor
broke through the skin, causing a gaping wound, which became infected.
The odor caused problems at work. Edna tried to conceal it with body
powder and cologne, which worked at first. Her kids started trying to get
her to come in and get help several months earlier, after a powerful, relentless stench finally set in.

Since Edna couldn't pay for private insurance and have enough money
left over to provide for her family, she had to come to Grady. Officially,
Grady treats any resident of the two counties that support it: Fulton and
DeKalb. When I arrived in Atlanta in 2001, the hospital was lax in en-
forcing the residency requirement. It ended up being the hospital for
poor people in many surrounding counties, even though only Fulton and
DeKalb taxpayers paid. As costs grew, Grady was forced to require proof
of residency.

Our doctors are good, but free care comes at the cost of time lost waiting for appointments, waiting for tests. You can spend an entire day waiting for a service that a private doctor's office provides in fifteen minutes or
less. People like Edna, who need every day's earnings and who can easily
be jettisoned from their jobs, can afford time away from work even less
than professionals, who may have some savings and job security. So people
like Edna wait until it's impossible to wait any longer; they come to see us
when it's too late.

* * *

WHY do black women end up with more aggressive breast cancer? Is this due to some biological characteristic that correlates with race, perhaps even determined by it? Can there be such a thing as white breast cancer and black breast cancer? Could these be different diseases?

You have to synthesize a pile of statistical data and medical literature to get insight into these problems, but it's worth the effort: You end up with extraordinarily valuable insights into the epidemiology and biology of cancer. More than that, you gain insight into economic structures in our society and, ultimately, something very big: the meaning of race.

At a glance, breast cancer in a black woman like Edna appears to differ from breast cancer in an average white woman. If you plot breast cancer on a spectrum from the worst prognosis to the best, a higher proportion of black women would wind up on the worst end.

One of the most ominous varieties of breast cancer is called triple-negative, because it is immune to three commonly used treatments. The surface of the cancer cell in that form of the disease lacks receptors to the hormones estrogen and progesterone and is similarly devoid of receptors to the HER-2/neu protein.

We have drugs that target breast cancer through these three channels. However, in triple-negative breast cancer, these drugs have nothing to latch onto, and all we can do is resort to desperate measures: harsher chemotherapies, which we know are frequently of little or no use.

About 30 percent of breast cancer in black women is triple-negative disease, compared to 18 percent in white women.

This disparity could appear to suggest a biological difference, but in fact it's rooted in cultural, historical, and societal divides. To understand this, we have to look at the potential causes of breast cancer in white and black women.

To start with, let's consider the incidence of better-prognosis cancer among white women. Instead of asking why black women are more likely to get more virulent breast cancer, let's ask why white women are more likely to develop the disease that has a better prognosis.

The answer can be gleaned in part from the incidence statistics.

For the past three decades—or for as long as we have had a national registry—the incidence of breast cancer has been higher in white women than in black women.

In 2000, the National Cancer Institute's Surveillance, Epidemiology, and End Results registry reported that during the previous year, blacks had an age-adjusted incidence rate of 125 per 100,000 women. In the past twenty years, the black incidence rate has bounced between the low of 105 per 100,000 in 1989 to the high point of 126 in 2008.

In 2000, white women had an incidence rate of 143 per 100,000. The breast cancer incidence rate in whites had risen from the 1970s, peaked at 147 per 100,000 in 1999, and has fallen to 129 per 100,000 in 2008.

The incidence rates were substantially apart over the past couple of decades, but have now nearly evened out. Was this occurring because white women were using mammography more and were therefore more likely to get diagnosed?

Not quite. The proportion of women getting mammography screening is roughly the same among whites and blacks. (I suspect that the proportion getting high-quality mammography is greater among whites than blacks, but this difference has not been adequately studied.)

The delay of pregnancy and childbirth is a more plausible explanation. White women tend to have children later in life than black women. Professional women, regardless of their race, go to college, establish their careers, and then have kids. Delaying childbirth past the age of thirty clearly increases the risk of breast cancer. To be specific, it increases the risk of estrogen-receptor-positive breast cancer, which has a better prognosis.

Also, white women have been more likely to use postmenopausal hormone-replacement therapy (HRT). Doctors prescribed HRT because it made sense logically. Without definitive data on the therapy's biological effect, doctors were, in effect, staging a decades-long societal experiment.

By 2003, 35 percent of postmenopausal white American women had taken this therapy at some time. For cultural and socioeconomic reasons, black women tended not to take HRT. Fewer than 5 percent of postmenopausal black women took HRT. This is important, because HRT is associated with better prognosis breast cancer.

In 2003, an analysis from the well-designed study called the Women's

Health Initiative showed that HRT was correlated with an increased risk of breast cancer. It was actually correlated with an increased risk of estrogen-receptor-positive, better prognosis breast cancer. The societal experiment was over.

The analysis led to a drop in the use of HRT, which likely accounts for the drop in breast cancer in white women from 147 per 100,000 in 1999 to 129 per 100,000 in 2008.

A focus on some geographic areas offers insight into what drives breast cancer in educated white women.

Consider Long Island. The area has been known to have a higher incidence of breast cancer than among the general United States population.

In the early 1990s, breast cancer advocates petitioned the U.S. Congress to force the National Cancer Institute to study the "high rates of breast cancer in Nassau and Suffolk Counties on Long Island." This led to Public Law 103-43, which prompted a series of studies, called the Long Island Breast Cancer Study Project.

At the beginning of the project, the incidence of breast cancer among Long Island's white women was 138.7 per 100,000 in Nassau County and 142.7 per 100,000 in Suffolk, compared to 127.8 per 100,000 in the United States as a whole.

Mortality from breast cancer on Long Island wasn't especially elevated. Indeed, several areas of New York State and many areas of the United States had higher death rates. A similarly high incidence was found among white women in the area north of San Francisco Bay.

Could the elevated incidence have been due to electromagnetic fields, hazardous wastes, or some other environmental cause?

After spending at least $20 million, the Long Island study project did not identify any pollutant that could be responsible for the elevated incidence of breast cancer.

However, those who believed that an environmental factor was at play were right. At least two such factors were driving the disparity between Long Island and the rest of the country: a higher level of education among area women and their choice to delay childbirth.

*   *   *

LET's return to the disparity in triple-negative breast cancer by race: 30 percent in black breast cancer patients, and 18 percent in white patients.

There is no difference in the proportion of black and white women with progesterone-positive or HER2-positive disease. So if we are to focus on the 12 percent disparity, we must look exclusively at the racial difference in the prevalence of the estrogen receptor.

Does *this* suggest that skin color stands for some biological difference? Not really.

Because of dietary differences that are caused by culture and socioeconomic status, a black girl in the United States accumulates weight much faster than a white girl. In the 1960s, the Centers for Disease Control and Prevention compared the start of menstruation by age. The study showed that the average age of menarche for white American girls was 12.8 years. For black American girls, it was 12.4 years. This is a bigger difference than it might seem. It means that 53 percent of black girls have started menstruating by their thirteenth birthday, compared to 43 percent of white girls.

Body mass index, a calculation based on weight and height, correlates with early nutrition status, which has a lot to do with age at first menstruation. Poor Americans have diets higher in calories and reach the weight of one hundred pounds faster.

Just the simple number of uninterrupted menstrual cycles increases the risk of breast cancer later in life.

The reason for this rapid weight gain in black girls has nothing to do with race, but reflects a high caloric intake and a diet rich in carbohydrates, a socioeconomic determinant of health. It's not about race. It's at least in part about the sort of food that is available in poor areas of inner cities.

The area of Detroit where I grew up and the areas of Atlanta where my patients come from are known as produce deserts. Grocery stores there carry all the chips, sodas, and mentholated cigarettes you may desire, but if you want a head of lettuce, you are out of luck.

You observe the same problems among poor whites, yet you don't see them among wealthy, well-educated blacks.

I cite the CDC data from the 1960s because they measure the racial differences that are driving breast cancers we are diagnosing today. This disparity has since widened, and if we trace it, we can project the differences in breast cancer rates and prevalence of triple-negative disease for decades into the future.

This extrapolation produces a deeply disturbing picture: the black-white gap in the onset of menstruation and body weight has dramatically widened, which means that the disease disparities will widen also.

FOR the sake of argument, let's set aside everything we know about Grady, Atlanta, and our race-obsessed society. Perhaps the best way to learn about breast cancer is to look at Scotland.

Scotland, which is virtually all-white, collects data at its every-ten-year census using a unique tool called the deprivation index. The index measures socioeconomic factors beyond household income. It asks about indoor plumbing, electricity, even how many servants one might employ. This index can discern that a college philosophy professor earning $55,000 per year is in a different socioeconomic stratum from a garbage collector earning $70,000 per year.

Using this index, a group of researchers found evidence pointing to a correlation between social deprivation and incidence of breast cancer that lacks estrogen receptors, a characteristic which makes the disease harder to treat. The deprived or poor who developed breast cancer were more likely to develop this kind of breast cancer. I find it ironic that one of the most important studies in minority health was an all-white study.

My friend Samuel Broder, when he was the director of the National Cancer Institute, used to say that poverty is a carcinogen. Skin color can be a marker of some sort, but you have to be careful not to rely on it too heavily. Wealth is a marker, too, as is education. Area of geographic origin and family history are also important, and all these factors must be considered.

EDNA has Stage IV breast cancer. Disease has spread all over her body. Had she come to see me early in the course of her disease, it would have cost about $30,000 to cure her. She could have remained a taxpayer. Her kids could have had a mother. Now, the cure is not an option. Still, we'll fight. We will give her breast-cancer chemotherapy that will cost more than $150,000, even though the chances are she will still die in less than two years. If you are a caring doctor, you realize she is just fifty-three, with kids and folks who love her, and your motivation is akin to a philosophy of Wayne Gretzky: "You miss every shot you don't take."

Every time I start chemo for metastatic disease I think of a patient named Sandra, a lively, young black woman whom I have treated for six years. She had brain metastases when I first met her. She has had active disease ever since, and even the doctor who sent her to me reminds me every time he sees me that he is amazed that she is alive, functional, and enjoying life.

Yes, sometimes cancer drugs give us "long-term survival," in the dispassionate language of those of us who study outcomes. But for every Sandra, we get fifty patients with metastatic disease who "don't do well." They live a median eighteen months, which means that half are living and half are dead a year and a half after diagnosis.

We try three treatments and contain Edna's disease for a while. She dies at age fifty-five, about twenty months after walking into the ER.

Chapter 2

Brawleyism

MY GREAT-GREAT-GRANDFATHER Edward McKnight Brawley was a free Negro born in Charleston, South Carolina. In the 1880s, Edward, who was a Baptist minister and author of a textbook on evangelism, moved his family to Selma, Alabama, to become president of Selma University, an all-black school.

His son Benjamin became one of the premier black intellectuals of his generation. He was educated at Morehouse College, Harvard University, and—like me—the University of Chicago.

Benjamin was the dean of Morehouse and later the chairman of the English Department at Howard. He was a literary critic, poet, writer, historian, and sociologist. A building at Morehouse is called Brawley Hall. There is a Brawley High School in Scotland Neck, North Carolina. He was quoted by his peers, including the historian W. E. B. DuBois in his treatise *Black Reconstruction in America*.

A biographer describes Benjamin as an intellectual inclined "to move simply as an American citizen in a democratic society." Liberal arts education and cultural advancement were his weapons of choice in the struggle for the rights of the Negro people.

In the thirties, the writers and literary critics of the Harlem Renaissance turned my great-uncle's name into a disparaging political moniker: *Brawleyism*. To a movement fueled by jazz, outrage, and the politics of the left, Benjamin seemed bourgeois. While his detractors expressed themselves in an unrestrained manner, Benjamin wrote Victorian verse and uplifting biographies of black Americans who were as worthy of admiration as the founding fathers. Benjamin's 1937 book, *Negro Builders and Heroes*, for example, profiles Frederick Douglass, Harriet Tubman, Sojourner Truth, and Booker T. Washington. A section is also devoted to his father, my great-great-grandfather.

Benjamin fought back, accusing his critics of excessive emphasis on the experience of the underclass and overlooking stories of triumph against the odds.

I admire people on both sides of that debate, and I don't side with either Benjamin or his detractors. There is no need to choose. The experience of the underclass cannot be ignored, yet there is no reason to diminish the achievements of Negro builders and heroes.

I view this half-forgotten schism of the pre-civil-rights era in the broader context of a continuum of human struggle against injustice, which goes beyond race and encompasses basic human rights, including the right to decent health care. The debate is raging still, and as chief medical officer of the American Cancer Society I list myself among its participants.

In this debate, I consider myself more fortunate than Benjamin Brawley. My form of Brawleyism plays out in science, which—unlike literary criticism—can produce measurable, reproducible results.

THIS book is a guided tour of the back rooms of American medicine. When I was fresh out of the University of Chicago medical school and newly admitted behind the curtains of these back rooms, I could dismiss medical horror stories as isolated episodes of the malfunctioning of the system: another person overlooked, another judgment error, another example of bum luck, another case of the frustratingly slow march of progress.

More than a quarter century later, I have seen enough to conclude that no incident of failure in American medicine should be dismissed as an aberration. Failure *is* the system, and those of us who are not yet its victims are at high risk of being sucked into its turbines.

My friend and colleague Peter Bach is fond of saying, "America does not have a health-care system. We have a sick-care system." Peter, a health-systems researcher and a pulmonologist at Memorial Sloan-Kettering Cancer Center, goes on to say that it's a stretch to use the word *system* to describe our health care because this word denotes organization.

Too often, helping the patient isn't the point. Economic incentives can dictate that the patient be ground up as expensively as possible with the goal of maximizing the cut of every practitioner who gets involved. When we, doctors, are at our best, we set aside our self-interest and put the patient's interest first. When we aren't at our best, the public pays more in fees, insurance premiums, taxes—and poor outcomes.

I get furious every time I hear politicians and pundits assert that the American health-care system is the best in the world. I heard this far too often from opponents of the 2010 health-care reform bill. I can think of several explanations for repeating this falsehood. Ignorance is the first and most elegant. Being out of touch with reality would explain it, as would lying, either to ourselves or to others.

America is the greatest place in the world to get care for a complicated but treatable disease if you have the ability to get the care and pay for it. It's not a great place to be sick if you are poor and uninsured or want consistent, basic care.

When you look at outcomes, our health-care system—technology notwithstanding—is closer to Communist states, both former and current, than to other technologically advanced nations.

The CIA publishes a lot of information that is publically available. The agency's data notes that life expectancy for Americans is 78.37 years. This makes us No. 50 among nations. Taiwan is No. 51. Monaco is on top, with the life expectancy of 89.73 years. Canada is No. 12, with 81.3 years, the United Kingdom is No. 28, with 80.05 years.

Some argue that this comparison is inappropriate since the United States has high homicide and accident rates compared to other first-world countries. I argue that this is the very point. Homicide, accident prevention, and other preventive health measures are a part of the health-care system and are recognized as such by most outside this country.

Life expectancy is heavily driven by infant mortality rates. This is not an area where we have much to be proud of. Forty-four countries have better infant mortality rates than the United States, including Cuba and Slovenia. This means that compared to a lot of other countries—many of them vastly poorer than us—we have a problem getting good care to pregnant women and babies.

And we pay a lot for mediocre results. Per capita, our health-care spending is the highest in the world. Here we are, indeed, No. 1. The No. 2 slot belongs to Switzerland, but our spending exceeds theirs by 50 percent. Americans spend two and a half times more on health care than on food.

Health care's share of America's gross domestic product is expanding. It jumped to 17.3 percent in 2009 from 16.2 percent in 2008—the largest single-year increase since 1960. At the current rate of growth, health-care costs are predicted to jump to $4.5 trillion in 2019.

At that point, health care will account for 19.3 percent—almost a fifth—of our gross domestic product. Some estimate that these increases are on course to make health care account for 25 percent of our economy by 2025.

Conservative pundits and politicians are fond of maligning the Canadian health-care system. Yet, Canadians spend half of what we do per capita. Switzerland is ranked tenth in life expectancy, and Canada is seventh. As No. 50 and the biggest spender by far, we aren't getting what we pay for.

Efforts to slow the expansion of our health-care system predate my career in medicine. Twenty-five years after I earned my white coat, from all my vantage points—as a doc on the ward, as an epidemiologist, and as a policy-maker—I see the same picture: our medical system fails to provide care when care is needed and fails to stop expensive, often unnecessary, and frequently harmful interventions even in situations when science proves these interventions are wrongheaded.

From my vantage points, I see that one painfully obvious approach to health-care reform has never been tried: No one has tried to make the entire system function rationally, based on science.

I devote a lot of time to studying the huge disparities in outcomes observed in the United States. *Disparities in outcome* is a euphemism for needless suffering and needless deaths. And these disparities in health results are often linked to the ability to pay.

In the back rooms of American medicine, the analysis of the patient's financial durability has a glib name: *a wallet biopsy*. If it returns positive, you stay in the hospital, you get more treatment, you can make a follow-up appointment. If it returns negative, you have little hope of getting consistent care.

Off the top, the wallet biopsy denies quality health care to the almost 51 million Americans who have no insurance. Often they get care of appalling quality or no care at all until they become sick enough or old enough for government benefits to kick in. As soon as this happens, the system welcomes them as sources of revenue, because even at Medicare and Medicaid coverage rates, you can make money on uncontrolled diabetes, kidney failure, heart disease, and late-stage cancer.

Here's a secret: wealth in America is no protection from getting lousy care. Wealth can increase your risk of getting lousy care. I spend a lot of time explaining to wealthy, insured patients that treatments they are convinced they need can't be expected to make them live longer or better lives. (In the following pages I will describe many such conversations.) When wealthy patients demand irrational care, it's not hard to find a doctor willing to provide it. If you have more money, doctors sell you more of what they sell, and they just might kill you.

It's regrettable that the most recent round of debates over health-care reform focused on alleged threats to ration health care—that "death panels" would be formed to save money on caring for the rich and spend it on caring for the poor was an effective scare tactic. People who scream about the rationing of health care fail to mention that rationing is already happening. My colleagues and I, all good doctors, are always arguing with health insurance companies that want to reduce costs by telling us we cannot perform a particular test or use a particular treatment.

Opponents of health-care reform have misstated our national dilemma. Health care is being rationed, while at the same time, irrational spending on unproven care is rampant.

I am not especially concerned about the rationing of health care. I am more concerned about something else entirely: rational use of health care.

The problem is, we don't use our expensive drugs and technologies appropriately. Instead of using these interventions to benefit patients, we use them to maximize revenues, and often harm patients. If we could learn to practice medicine rationally, the money we would save would help us provide the most basic care for those who are now shut out of the system. Health care for the rich would benefit as well, because in medicine gluttony equals harm.

A rational system of health care has to have the ability to say no, and to have it stick. This is the only way to protect patients from misguided, scientifically unproven interventions, to cut out waste, fraud, and abuse. Those who pay—private insurers or the government—need to be able to protect the public from the miscarriage of medicine.

Denying useless treatment needn't be motivated by saving money. Let's focus on not doing harm, refraining from peddling snake oil and false hope. I empathize with a patient who views an unproven procedure as her only hope for living longer, but I have nothing but contempt for a medical practitioner who labels bullshit "hope" and profits handsomely from it.

It's possible to provide better care at a lower price. It's possible to be justly proud of our scientific and technological achievements and provide quality and consistent primary care.

It's possible to have innovation and quality and access and lower costs. There is no need to choose.

I am not worried about breaking ranks. I look forward to it.

Some of my colleagues are willing to play the game, realizing that care—even useless and inappropriate care—makes cash registers emit pleasing sounds. We doctors are paid for services we provide, a variant of "piecework" that guarantees that we will err on the side of selling more, sometimes believing that we are helping, sometimes knowing that we are not, and sometimes simply not giving a shit.

Would a doctor who sells radiation therapy tell you to go across the street to get chemotherapy, even in cases where studies show that it's more appropriate? Would either of these medical entrepreneurs advise you to wait for six months to see whether your disease is of the sort that would actually harm you? All too often, the answers to these questions are no.

The financial incentives that drive the medical community have a devastating impact on patients and health-care costs, and we will not change unless we are forced to change. Doctors who own labs have been shown to order more tests than doctors who don't. A doctor at a for-profit practice is more likely to prescribe the treatments that benefit him the most. I've heard of community oncology practices that hold regular meetings to inform doctors about treatment techniques that maximize billing.

When money is to be made, the system can be proactive, again to the detriment of the patient. Call it "disease mongering" or call it the marketing of disease, but as I write this, a fleet of aquamarine, white, and blue mobile homes is bringing prostate cancer screening to a shopping-mall parking lot near you. These things are long, thirty-nine feet, plenty of room. Come aboard! The blood test is free, but the cascade of follow-up services will ring up considerable sales for treatments that leave guys impotent and incontinent. Treatment that *may* have a minuscule chance of saving them from cancer, but have a much larger chance of treating a cancer that would never have harmed them, or may not even have been there in the first place.

Improvements in health come at a cost, but in the case of prostate cancer, no one has shown an improvement in mortality. Despite concerted efforts, screening for prostate cancer has not been clearly proven to decrease men's chances of dying of prostate cancer. But that doesn't mean there isn't money to be made; recently, I noticed that Zero, an advocacy group that operates these screening vans, receives funding from the makers of Depend diapers.

I know doctors who are just plain bad. Why do they continue to practice without impediment? The answer is simple: because no one is looking over their shoulders, no one files a disciplinary complaint, no tribunal of peers punishes them unless they do something spectacularly awful. No one is better suited to police the profession than the profession itself. But our professional societies tend to choose misguided collegiality over the well-being of our patients, the people who trust us with their lives.

I will show how we academic physicians who practice in nonprofit institutions such as Emory are not pristine either. If you don't watch out, we'll sell you on a clinical trial that will get our names on scientific papers, but not necessarily be appropriate for your disease. Even as academics, we may be motivated to maximize billing to support our departments. Or we may simply be enthusiastic about the procedures and therapies we are trained to deliver.

It's not easy to challenge doctors to justify their decisions in the clinic. As we'll see, it's harder still to challenge a wrongheaded consensus of a medical specialty as it marches in lockstep. This is precisely what happens when professional societies of doctors who perform expensive medical procedures issue "evidence-based guidelines" that are anything but evidence-based guidelines. Instead, the purpose of many of these documents is to protect the specialties' financial stake in the system.

Why not just say no to the special-interest groups that peddle interventions that generate billions while doing harm?

Why not center the system on benefiting the patient, not the people who profit from lying to the patient?

Why not set realistic, scientifically based goals for treating our patients?

Why not teach doctors to start using the simple words *I don't know*?

Why not teach doctors and insurers to say no to patients who are determined to get care that has no scientific basis?

Why not stop treatment when—scientifically, based on evidence—there is nothing left to do?

IF the wreckage of health-care reforms attempted over the past twenty-five years is an indication, change from above will not get the job done.

Yet, high-quality health care for all is as much a civil rights issue as is one man, one vote. In health care—as in voting rights—real change will have to come from below, not only from patients, but from all of us as citizens.

Sadly, patients who understand the system are a small, politically insignificant minority. The majority is placid at best, confused at worst. Many patient groups act as unquestioning advocates for pharmaceutical companies and medical specialties, failing to realize that the interests for which they advocate run counter to their own.

In the most recent round of reform, we saw special-interest groups of all sorts coming to the defense of their entitlements. It was hard not to notice the opponents of change, but if there was even a trace of a public movement on the part of proponents of change, I missed it entirely. Political moderates and progressives remained silent even as debates became dominated by Tea Party conservatives and fictional characters created by PR firms on behalf of business interests.

Proponents of science as a foundation for health care have not come together to form a grassroots movement, and until this happens, all of us will have to live with a system built on pseudoscience, greed, myths, lies, fraud, and looking the other way.

Patients need to understand that more care is not better care, that doctors are not necessarily right, and that some doctors are not even truthful.

Genuine health-care reform—like the right to vote—will not be granted magnanimously. Like civil rights, the right to good health care will have to be won in public struggle. To bring about real change, real people will have to say, "Enough!"

I draw on the best source of information available to me as a physician: patients. What role did the health-care system play in their disease? Have my colleagues made treatment decisions based on the patients' interests or based on self-interest? Have I been able to mitigate harm, or have I caused it? How have we doctors caused harm? Through uninformed but billable trial and error? By denying care? By providing the wrong care, or too much care?

Although the stories in this book are true, names and identifying characteristics of patients have been changed to protect their privacy, except in cases where individual patients went public with their struggles. The names and identifying characteristics of physicians have also been changed to protect their privacy, except where I discuss their scientific publications. In clinical anecdotes, I note when doctors are identified by their real names.

The views expressed here are not those of the American Cancer Society or Emory University.

And, of course, the views expressed by the authors of this book are not intended as a substitute for medical advice, diagnosis, or treatment provided by the reader's personal physicians.

Chapter 3

Cadillac Care

WHY DO I WORK at Grady?

To do some good, if I can.

That's part of my motivation, but not all of it. I go to Grady for reasons that wouldn't surprise my grandfather Willie Brawley. Willie, Benjamin's nephew, was a sharecropper.

I can see that in 1930 a man whose name matches my grandfather's was listed among inmates at the Wetumpka State Prison in Alabama. It could be him. According to a family story, he became a union organizer and was lynched in 1948. My family didn't treat his death as something to be proud of. Even my grandmother—his wife, whom I knew well—didn't talk about him much.

As a black man and a union organizer in the South, he surely understood what he was up against. Apparently nothing beckons a Brawley more powerfully than a hopeless cause, and I hear its call on the PA system at Grady. I go to Grady to understand where we are betraying our patients, where we are betraying ourselves, and how we can learn to do better. If you want to stay grounded, Grady is the place.

Respect for people I knew growing up in Detroit could be a part of it, too. As I grow older and more experienced, I become increasingly amazed by the wisdom of those folks. When you are black and poor, you are by definition a survivor, and survivors have reasons to be suspicious. My parents and their friends didn't trust doctors, didn't trust hospitals. A hospital was the place where they withheld treatment or where

29

they tried things on you without telling you what they were doing and why.

White doctors think that we—black folks—worry about becoming unwitting subjects of medical experiments. That's not quite it. Folks I grew up with were worried that the doctors who treated them had no idea what they were doing, that they were experimenting, trying various drugs or treatments, hoping that something might finally work. My family members were afraid they would pay the price for exercises in trial and error. It was about trust.

When I was starting my career in medicine, I was contemptuous of such thinking. Initially, I dismissed these folks as outsiders who were suspicious of the system that excluded them. Now, having seen the way medicine is commonly practiced, I see that they were right to be suspicious.

Now I wonder, can all of us benefit from a dose of skepticism? Can the health-care system make itself trustworthy, become accessible and driven by science?

I begin my search for answers at Grady, where patients are vulnerable, contrasts stark, lessons harsh. Yet, these are not entirely stories of desperation. Since we take patients no one wants, and without expectation of payment, we are immune to market pressures and the plethora of perverse incentives that spread dysfunction through the health-care system.

Thus shielded, we can—often—provide better care than doctors who treat the rich. Also, any care provided at Grady has to be based on solid evidence. I am not suggesting that Grady is perfect. It has many flaws that come with underfunding, and many challenges that come from caring for the uninsured. Yet, at Grady, an effort to disregard science will be shot down fast.

The technical term for millions of people like Edna Riggs is the *underserved*. Edna didn't receive medical care until the manifestations of her disease became catastrophic. Another of my breast cancer patients—Helen Williams—started out on the opposite end of this scale. She had the most advanced care Atlanta had to offer.

*   *   *

IN 1990, Helen, then fifty, finds a lump in her breast. Without delay, she goes to her gynecologist, who sends her to get a mammogram. The tumor can't be seen on the image, but the gynecologist does the right thing. He refers Helen to Luther Smith, one of the best-known breast-cancer surgeons in the Southeast.

Smith performs a needle biopsy, which leads to the diagnosis of breast cancer. The tumor looks aggressive under the microscope. Though scared, Helen reminds herself of her good fortune. She is married, her kids are grown, her job benefits at a financial-services company include excellent health insurance, and she is discerning enough to demand the best treatment modern medicine can provide.

The tumor turns out to be four centimeters in its maximum size— quite large. Altogether, twenty-one lymph nodes are resected, and all prove negative. This means that the disease may not have spread. The biology of the tumor is worrisome. It's estrogen- and progesterone-receptor negative, meaning hormonal therapies cannot be used. Hers is the sort of high-grade, aggressive disease that is more likely to occur in black women than in white women. This mixed bag of good and bad characteristics translates into the diagnosis of Stage II disease.

Helen is offered a choice of surgical procedures: a lumpectomy and radiation or a mastectomy. She chooses mastectomy. The insurance company doesn't object. The company also pays a plastic surgeon to rebuild the breast. She is offered postsurgical chemotherapy. Insurance agrees to pay for this, too.

This scary time has a special meaning for Helen, who had witnessed the civil rights movement and integration transform Atlanta in the sixties, seventies, and eighties. Here she is, a black woman in the South, getting Cadillac care. She feels fortunate.

Smith, the surgeon, refers Helen to his favorite medical oncologist, Norman Kuhn, who is known for an especially aggressive approach to treating breast cancer. The oncologist explains that a stronger dose of chemo is better than a weaker dose. "More is better" has been a hallmark of the oncology profession since the 1950s: the more chemotherapy you administer to the patient, the more effective it is in terms of killing the disease.

Kuhn has treated a lot of breast cancer, and he favors a take-no-prisoners technique for "adjuvant"—postsurgical—therapy. This is a procedure in which we give chemotherapy drugs after surgery to eradicate cancer that was too small to be seen by the naked eye in the surgical area, or too small to be seen with radiological imaging if it has spread to the distant organs, including the liver, the lungs, and the brain.

The oncologist's plan for Helen's treatment seems logically compelling: a high dose of drugs will be used to kill all the cancer cells that might be hiding in her body. The doses will be so high that the bone marrow—an innocent bystander—will be destroyed. It used to be that this much chemo would kill the patient, but no longer. Doctors had recently developed an ingenious technique that enabled them to take the patient to the brink of death from chemotherapy, then—at the last moment—rescue her. To save Helen from succumbing to the toxic effects of chemotherapy, her own bone marrow will be harvested and stored before chemotherapy and reinjected after the drugs complete their work. This procedure is called autologous bone marrow transplantation.

Again, Helen feels fortunate to be treated by the best in the South. These are doctors with impeccable credentials and reputations. Would they have treated a black woman fifteen or twenty years earlier? Now they treat her like any other patient. She enjoys their courteous treatment—and she trusts them.

Kuhn explains that Helen's insurance will pay for most of the cost of the transplant and chemotherapy. The procedure requires hospitalization, but it's usually just for a few days. There will be some side effects. Helen will lose her hair, but it will grow back. She might feel tired for a while, and the risk of infections will be increased. All of this seems to be a small price to pay for the security that comes with Kuhn's promise to make the cancer go away forever.

Given these arguments and that she and her husband trust the doctors and are satisfied with the care they are receiving, Helen agrees to the transplant.

Helen checks into a private hospital, which she knows didn't integrate until 1980. There, she is taken to the OR and given general anaesthesia. She wakes up three hours later with a bandage over her upper buttocks and her bone marrow harvested. It will come to the rescue after the chemotherapy eradicates the disease.

Helen returns to the hospital ten days later, after some wound healing. High-dose chemo is about to start. She is put in a private room where no flowers or raw vegetables are allowed. (They might have infectious agents on them.) The next morning, a central line is inserted into the subclavian vein in her right upper chest.

Helen and the nurse starting the first infusion joke about how this feels similar to an execution by lethal injection. However, Helen quickly reminds herself that the cocktail of poisons she is about to receive will kill the cancer, not her.

Infusions cause unease. Even twenty-four hours after treatment ends, she has nausea. Five days after getting the chemotherapy, it has washed out of her system. Her white blood cell count and platelet count start to fall. The harvested bone marrow is thawed and infused into her subclavian vein.

The side effects Helen experiences are far more severe than she expected. She is unable to recall most of them having been described to her prior to the procedure. She has nausea, vomiting, diarrhea, dehydration. Her marrow is slow to reimplant and start producing. She has bleeding caused by a low platelet count and severe anemia. She has both gastrointestinal bleeding and bleeding from the incisions made to harvest her bone marrow. She has mouth and gum problems. She has cardiac-rhythm problems. She has a change in mental status due to electrolyte imbalances. She has a respiratory arrest and is put on a ventilator. She develops pneumonia. She has a tracheotomy. Altogether she spends five months in a hospital, only to be discharged to a rehab hospital. Helen survives it all and returns to work nearly a year after leaving for the bone marrow transplant.

Three years after her discharge, she reads a news story about randomized clinical trials that showed that bone marrow transplantation for breast cancer doesn't prolong survival.

At her next scheduled appointment, Helen brings up the trial results with her oncologist, Kuhn. Yes, the results are disappointing, the oncologist concedes. Though he still believes that transplants are beneficial in some cases, he is no longer performing the procedure, he says. Mostly, he stopped because the media has unnecessarily scared the patients, and insurance companies are declining to pay.

Helen asks whether her transplant had been performed as part of the clinical trials that showed that the procedure didn't work. Being part of the group of women who helped science learn the truth would have made her suffering worthwhile, Helen reasons. It wouldn't be too different from getting clubbed in a civil rights march.

No, says Kuhn. He didn't participate in trials.

This is abrupt and puzzling. Why had she been subjected to a devastating procedure when no one—including her doctor—could say with certainty whether it worked? Why wasn't she told about this uncertainty? As far as she could recall, Dr. Kuhn sounded quite certain of his facts when he described the procedure. Was it possible that she was duped? Was it possible that she had nearly died to help her doctor and various Atlanta medical institutions accumulate wealth? More important, why hadn't she been told the procedure was unproven?

"Why did we do this?" she asks Kuhn.

"This was what everybody was doing at the time," he responds.

This answer is more or less correct. Many breast-cancer patients and their physicians had been unwilling to take chances on anything less than a transplant. They thought that more would automatically mean better. Fundamental scientific questions—such as determining whether the procedure was beneficial—were conveniently sidestepped in the day-to-day practice of medicine.

The amounts of money that could be made by doctors and hospitals didn't foster skepticism. Each transplant procedure cost at least $150,000 when it became commercially available. Later, the price was knocked down to about $60,000, roughly the price of a luxury car. Complicated cases such as Helen's were worth $1 million or more in medical services.

As the government was trying to control aggregate health-care costs, hospitals were finding that transplant programs were allowing them to recoup some of the lost revenues. Since the transplanters were using approved drugs in a new way, the Food and Drug Administration didn't need to be consulted.

It was a fine business opportunity, and one company—Nashville-based Response Oncology Inc.—offered to set up transplant programs at community hospitals. Setting up the program required a few hundred thousand dollars and a few days of training, but the payback was nearly immediate.

Regardless of whether they received transplants at Dana-Farber Cancer Institute or at a hospital down the street, patients were largely convinced that the approach worked, and many of them sued insurers for any effort to restrict coverage. For years, well-meaning people throughout the United States held community bake sales and charity raffles to raise money for a bone marrow transplantation for a breast-cancer patient in their midst. These friends and neighbors had no idea that they were helping some doctor get rich on an unproven procedure that harmed the patient.

The numbers of women who were unwittingly, unnecessarily—and, yes, fraudulently—harmed by this procedure is staggering. Between 1989 and 2001, at least twenty-three thousand women underwent the procedure outside clinical trials. Some estimates are much higher—thirty-five thousand to forty thousand.

Meanwhile, only a small number of American women—fewer than fifteen hundred—received this treatment in randomized clinical trials. These trials had a difficult time finding enough patients who were willing to take a chance of being assigned to standard treatment. Yet, after much hard work, the trials were completed and presented at the plenary session of the 1999 annual meeting of the American Society of Clinical Oncology in Atlanta.

Altogether, four randomized trials were presented. Three of them, conducted in the United States and Sweden, found that the procedure didn't improve survival. The fourth, conducted by Werner Bezwoda in South Africa, was remarkably positive. Alas, a year later that trial was found to be fraudulent.

I am proud to report that Grady didn't offer bone marrow transplants in breast cancer. We believed that transplants were unjustified as standard

care and should not be available outside well-designed, carefully monitored clinical trials.

HELEN is shaken by what she learns, but she continues to do well, and
that's what matters the most. She and her husband go out to dinner to
celebrate her fifth anniversary of being cancer-free. Even knowing what
she now knows, Helen doesn't feel betrayed by the medical profession.
She has suffered, sure, but she considers herself cured.

Four years later—nine years after the transplant—a routine chest
X-ray shows a lesion on Helen's lung. A CT-guided biopsy of the lung
shows something that looks like an adenocarcinoma, a slow-growing
form of lung cancer. A CT of the chest, abdomen, and pelvis and a nu-
clear medicine bone scan show this lesion as well. Is this lung cancer in a
nonsmoker, or has Helen's breast cancer returned despite the transplant?

The pathologist takes nearly two weeks to perform special stains and
even compares the tumor to her previous cancer. (This is possible because samples of her old tumor had been stored.) His conclusion: the
two-centimeter lesion is a metastasis. The breast cancer is back.

Helen's doctors bring up the possibility of removing a part of the lung
to extract this lesion. They say this might be the only lesion, in which
case the surgery might be curative. The decision is made to watch the
lesion for a few weeks. During this time, a second and third lesion appear in Helen's lungs. Clearly, this is inoperable metastatic disease. Now,
Helen's only hope is treatment that will prolong rather than save her life.

Shortly after the initial chest X-ray, Helen receives a registered letter
from her insurance company. The letter informs her that she has exceeded
her lifetime maximum for health insurance and the company will pay no
more. Facing a recurrence of breast cancer, Helen is pronounced uninsurable. What are her options?

This middle-class woman who has done everything her doctors told
her to do and has been put through tremendous amounts of what is now
considered unnecessary treatment that almost killed her several times
and cost a year of her life suddenly finds herself uninsured and dying of
cancer.

Helen and her husband are earning salaries, which makes them unqualified for Medicaid. Should she quit her job? How much longer would she be able to work anyway? Should they get a divorce so she might qualify for Medicaid? What kind of doctors take Medicaid? Helen's previous doctors did not.

A secretary in the oncologist's office suggests that she go to Grady, the county hospital. Where poor people go.

I meet Helen at the breast clinic. Because of my habit of actually talking with patients, I am running late, significantly late. Helen exudes discomfort, distrust, and suspicion. These emotions are hard to hide, especially from clinicians, who sense them as acutely as dogs sense fear. Is she irritated at having to wait?

She is slim, around five foot five, and has salt-and-pepper hair trending toward salt. She wears a tweed suit, the sort a businesswoman would wear to work. Her husband is with her, paying close attention, but saying little. He is there for moral support—and as another set of eyes and ears.

I think that a couple with such a distinguished and dignified appearance must feel out of place in the clinic's waiting room. The cancer center is not as Spartan as the rest of Grady. It was built with $30 million in tobacco-settlement money, and as the center's founding director, I got to work with the architects. Our typical patients are very different from the Williamses. Some of them are disheveled, some appear not to have taken a bath for a few days, and many look very sick.

As we begin to go over Helen's history, she quickly explains that she used to be insured, but has lost insurance. I realize that she is really trying to explain why she is at a public hospital, seeing me.

At Grady, patients simply don't talk about payment via private insurance, Medicare, or Medicaid. I am the one who brings up the subject—rarely—only to ascertain that the patients have a way to obtain the medications I prescribe. If coverage or copayments are a problem, a social worker takes care of finding the money, and, if necessary, Grady picks up the tab. Some of us like not having to think about fees, coverage, and reimbursement. That's why we are able to recruit good doctors to work at Grady.

I sense something else in that examination room, something I have been aware of since childhood: a black patient's suspicion of black doctors.

MY uncle Fred, a construction worker with his own business and my only close relative with real money, used to say, "You are in trouble if your lawyer, your doctor, and your accountant are not Jewish." This belief is rooted in pre-civil-rights days. Doctors, especially black doctors you didn't know, were thought to be out to make money off you rather than to help you. Jewish doctors were perceived to be empathetic, compassionate, and educated. (Thankfully, Uncle Fred didn't live strictly by this belief. He financed a chunk of my medical education at the University of Chicago.)

Black patients' prejudice against black doctors endures, now more as a fear that you got where you are not by brains and rigorous training, but because of an affirmative action program. I've heard black patients make disparaging remarks about "the *Bakke* case," a 1978 U.S. Supreme Court ruling that limited reliance on affirmative action. Allan Bakke, the white plaintiff in the case, was trying to get into the University of California, Davis, medical school, but was denied admission because the school was taking minority candidates with lower scores.

We turn to Helen's treatment plan. She has maxed out on Adriamycin, one of the workhorses of breast-cancer treatment. She received so much of it in the transplant that an additional dose would likely cause congestive heart failure. Since Helen's disease lacks estrogen receptors, hormonal treatment isn't an option. "Just to be sure, we should repeat pathology," I suggest. "I have had the experience of other hospitals getting it wrong."

While we are at it, I suggest that we take a PET-CT scan, to see the extent of metastases. Thanks to the tobacco settlement, I have the best PET-CT scanner in Atlanta. It's a fantastic gizmo. It uses the same scanner to produce positron-emission tomography and computed-tomography images. This is great, because it combines PET's ability to register metabolic and biochemical activity with CT anatomical imaging. This allows you to see simultaneously what's going on and where it's happening.

I can see that Helen likes that I am not willing to accept another hospital's diagnosis. "Are you aware of the controversy surrounding autologous bone marrow transplantation?" she asks. She is testing me. Am I a happy-go-lucky fool who takes everything on faith, or is there a little rigor in my brain?

I like being questioned. People who ask questions of their doctor get a better understanding of what's going to happen to them and are better able to adhere to the prescribed treatment. They can bring out the best in their doctor. "Not only do I know about it, I lived it," I say. "I trained to be a bone marrow transplanter at the National Cancer Institute. All of us did transplantation then."

"Did you do it in breast cancer?"

"No. Only in lymphoma and leukemia. But we were training because we were all going to be millionaires working in breast cancer. Now, being a transplanter in breast cancer is like being a typewriter repairman."

"Typewriters actually worked."

"True, but repairing them is a skill that's no longer needed. There is actually more work for guys who make horseshoes."

"Are you familiar with Werner Bezwoda?"

I am indeed. Werner Bezwoda, one of the pioneers of bone marrow transplantation in breast cancer, had been reporting extraordinary successes treating primarily black women in South Africa. He was the principal investigator on one of the four randomized trials of bone marrow transplantation in breast cancer. I sat in the front row at the plenary session of the 1999 annual meeting of the American Society of Clinical Oncology, watching him present. He seemed calm; there was no twitching, no excessive blinking.

Alas, Bezwoda's data were fraudulent from start to finish. He had no research protocol, no set regimen. Apparently, he made up the data as he went along. Nonetheless, until the fraud was discovered, physicians all over the world were citing his results and charging insurers for the highly toxic Bezwoda Regimen outside clinical trials.

"Nine years ago, would you have offered me a transplant?" Helen asks.

"I wouldn't have, but I would have had no problem with it, if you agreed to take part in a clinical trial and if you understood the risks. Many people were suing their insurance companies demanding it, and many doctors were blinded by the fact that they made money off it."

Bone marrow transplantation seemed to make sense logically. Experts in the field felt it worked, so it had to be good. Patients bought into this logic and sued insurance companies to force payment for this therapy. Ten states passed laws making it impossible for insurers to deny payment.

Medicine is especially susceptible to this kind of jumping the gun in adopting new treatments. Surgeons performed disfiguring radical procedures called the Halsted mastectomies for more than seventy-five years because William Stewart Halsted said it was the right way to treat breast cancer. Since he was from Johns Hopkins, he had to be right. An academic physician could get fired for questioning the value of the Halsted mastectomy. It was deemed irresponsible.

It took an iconoclast—Bernie Fisher, a surgeon at the University of Pittsburgh—to stage a randomized clinical trial that demonstrated that a conservative procedure followed by radiation was equivalent to radical mastectomy.

Suddenly, I realize that the roots of Helen's mistrust run deeper than reliance on racial stereotypes. Perhaps she mistrusts me because of my affiliation with a charity hospital and because the color of my skin is the same as her own. But there is something else—something we share. Skepticism.

"Do you feel that the risks of bone marrow transplantation were explained to you?" I ask to make sure that my hunch is correct.

"Not as I look back at it."

"I am sorry. You should know that this is not how I operate. I tell people what I know, what I don't know, and what I believe, and I label it accordingly."

Clearly, Helen is a patient who appreciates honesty, a skeptic who allowed skepticism to lapse long enough to receive an unnecessarily toxic, unproven treatment without adequate consent.

Now, her skepticism is back, and it's an honor to validate it. I want her to trust me, I want her to give me a chance to do my best to extend her life.

A few days after I meet Helen, a fellow hands me her PET-CT scan. "It lit up like a Christmas tree," she says.

Indeed, the scan lights up bright, showing lesions in the spine, ribs, pelvis, lung, liver, and the opposite breast. I warn her to steer away from such comparisons. There is a difference between Peace on Earth and metastatic disease.

HELEN becomes my friend and, at times, my conscience. She helps shape many of my feelings toward health care, the health-care industry, and health-care reform. I take her to lunch with her breast-cancer-survivor friends. She crochets a portrait of me. It is one of my true prized possessions.

She joins Grady's efforts to reach out to women like Edna Riggs. A lot of women are treated for breast cancer at Grady. Indeed, more than 1 percent of all black Americans diagnosed with breast cancer each year get treatment here. Bringing them into the system requires creativity.

To open our doors wider, Helen helps create a breast-cancer outreach program to encourage discussion about the disease the older black ladies in whispering tones called the Big C. Helen and other black breast-cancer survivors go into Atlanta's inner city and tell their stories to anyone who will listen. They create a gospel choir of one hundred breast-cancer survivors. I can't imagine a more spiritually uplifting way to demonstrate that it's possible to survive breast cancer.

When we get together, we talk about things that matter: life, death.

Helen reminds me in so many ways of the folks who worked hard so I wouldn't end up on the slab. I tell her that when I turned thirty, my mother and I sat down to figure out what happened to the kids who grew up with me in the neighborhood. We limited ourselves to young men born two years before me and two years after. Of the twelve of us, only three got out of the neighborhood. The rest were either dead or serving life sentences for capital crimes.

Keeping me alive was a project that involved many people. There was Miss Asher, a petite, brown-haired woman who taught my kindergarten class at Harry B. Keidan Elementary School. I remember us sitting on the floor with legs crossed "like Indians." I didn't like sitting on the floor like an Indian. I complained about it a lot. It was uncomfortable.

But Miss Asher was the first person outside my immediate family to let me know that I had all I needed to make something of myself. There wasn't a single episode, no single telling anecdote. It was more profound than that. She engendered the feeling that I was worthy of her respect. Every day, she let me know that she would be upset if I ended up a thug or in jail. She made me feel that I was somebody, that I could do something. Even more, she made me feel that it was *expected* that I would do something positive. Miss Asher didn't stop with me. She encouraged my mother to find a way to send me to the nearby Catholic school, St. Cecilia, where I could get the attention and instruction in the fundamentals I needed to flourish. My parents ultimately agreed to tighten their belts and squeeze out the tuition, which was $50 a year when I enrolled in second grade.

Miss Asher's encouragement stoked my imagination. My family and their friends saw some potential in me and mobilized to help.

Uncle Fred, my mother's brother, was always there with a wad of crisp cash: "Here, buy a book."

My father worked as a janitor at the VA hospital in Dearborn and had a sideline business of running numbers, an illegal lottery, there. Miss Farris, a white nurse at the VA, talked to me whenever she stopped by to pay off her numbers debts. For my seventh birthday, Miss Farris gave me my first doctor kit. It had a microscope and a stethoscope.

My father's bookies, too, were eager to chip in.

They kept peeling off bills even after I went off to college: "Here is ten dollars. . . . Here is twenty dollars." One of the bookies gave me $100 for my eighth-grade graduation, a substantial sum in 1973. They knew I would not blow the money on reefer. I was a good bet.

HELEN and I talk about civil rights and social justice, too. I tell Helen about my hope that a genuine popular movement will form to make medicine accessible, driven by science, and trustworthy. I tell her that I realize that nothing short of another civil rights movement will do. "Everything else has been tried," I say.

"We need another Martin," she says.

It's a wish. When I hear it from people I respect, I counter that the civil rights movement was first and foremost about equality, but it was quickly focused on the most obvious rights: the right to sit wherever the hell you want on the bus and the right to vote.

"These rights are important, but the right to equality in health care is no less important, and it has been left behind," I reply. "This is tricky in part because it's not as clear—and not as much about race—as the bus regulations in Montgomery. You can hope and pray for someone like Martin. Meanwhile, we must do what we can." Then I add, "As you have, Helen."

We both know death is near, and I don't want to miss my chance to tell Helen how great a privilege it was to watch her rise above her deadly experience with Cadillac care, to cast away anger about her losses, to triumph over cynicism and mistrust and blossom into a genuine advocate.

Chapter 4

Skepticism

WHEN THE DISEASE GATHERS a momentum we can't break, Helen accepts that she is dying. One of my great privileges as a physician and as a human being comes when from her hospice bed Helen asks me to speak at her funeral.

I have it flowing good when that day comes. I want to make my speech good for her. I talk about all she overcame in her life, how she struggled, how she displayed good humor, how she helped other patients. How she learned about the problem of women ignoring breast masses, sometimes for years, and that she helped us found a choir of breast-cancer survivors to communicate health messages to the black community. How she counseled other breast cancer patients, most of whom were not as sick as she was, but who felt sorrier for themselves than she did. How she took seriously her responsibility to teach and motivate the medical students, residents, and fellows and even the old men of the department to give the best care we can in a compassionate way.

I don't mention how ashamed I am that medicine had used Helen. That she received a bone marrow transplant without being told all that was known about it, and, more important, all that was unknown. She got the transplant because she was insured and doctors could convert her suffering into cash. Maybe her original doctor simply failed to ask the fundamental question. Maybe he failed to be scientific. Maybe the money helped cloud his judgment.

A funeral is not the place to discuss intellectual dishonesty, malfeasance, and conflicts of interest in medicine.

MY parents met in Detroit and settled on Philadelphia Street, in the area called Black Bottom, the black part of downtown.

I was born on July 4, 1959. In February 1960, using the GI Bill, my parents bought a "two-family flat" at 4224 Burlingame, in a West Side neighborhood then mostly inhabited by the Jews and Catholics, most of whom worked for the Ford Motor Company.

My mother quit her job as a hospital cashier to take care of my two sisters and me. We were living on my father's earnings as a janitor at the Veterans Administration hospital in Dearborn, his sideline of running numbers, and his moonlighting as a furniture upholsterer. Also, we rented out the apartment upstairs to help make mortgage payments. This was my father's idea of security.

I remember a color television being delivered on a cold day in February 1963. This is one of my earliest memories. My mother was pregnant with my little sister at the time. It's a happy memory, an image of optimism, freshness, beginnings. Twelve two-family flats were on our block. We were the second black family to move in.

By moving to Burlingame, a street near the commercial hub of Dexter Avenue, my family joined the deadly cycle called Black Fright/White Flight. Yet, race is paradoxically absent from my childhood memories. It's possible that it was forced out by a more fundamental concept: safety.

The whites were not stupid and not necessarily bigoted. They were interested in their own preservation, and they fled the neighborhood because danger was real. By the time I was five, in 1964, I knew that people stole. I knew that people shot other people. I knew what reefer was. I knew that there was such a thing as heroin. I knew that drug violence raged outside and that I was not going to get sucked into it. It was not unusual to hear that a corpse had been found in an alley in our neighborhood. Murder was what happened when people didn't pay their drug debts.

My family didn't leave the house much because we worried about burglaries, and whenever we did leave, we left the light on so the house seemed occupied. Cars were stolen, car batteries were stolen, even schoolkids' book bags were stolen, just for the sake of stealing. Living in fear of violence was the only life I knew.

I would be nearly twenty, halfway through the University of Chicago, before I realized that I was no longer looking over my shoulder or preparing to drop to the ground to evade stray bullets. (It should be noted that Hyde Park isn't the safest place in America. It's surrounded by projects and guarded by what was then the third-largest police force in Illinois.)

In mid-September 1965, my mother brought me to a Catholic school called St. Cecilia, seven blocks down the street. The school had been in session for two weeks. Still, Sister Lorenzo, the principal, decided to let me in.

The sisters of the Immaculate Heart of Mary, who ran the school, scared me at first. They walked like pelicans and wore dresses that hid their shoes. In the middle of my second year, in the spirit of the Second Ecumenical Council (Vatican II), the nuns were allowed to shorten their dresses by two inches, and we learned that they wore funny black, lace-up shoes.

It didn't take me long to realize that they were exceptionally kind women whose purpose in life was to give kids like me the means to achieve. My wife disagrees when I say this, but in many respects I think of nuns as the first women's libbers. They ran schools and hospitals when women didn't run any other major organizations. My respect for the nuns as authority figures influences me to this day as I see women in positions of authority that they did not have just a generation ago.

Miss Asher and I remained in contact even after she prevailed on my parents to enroll me in St. Cecilia. At least twice a year through sixth grade, my mother would drive me to the public school, where Miss Asher and I would spend time talking about things I could do, things I would do. I suspect that these meetings were arranged behind the scenes, with Miss Asher extending invitations or my mother making appointments. This was a shot of encouragement, and it was effective.

I loved Catholicism: the structure, the pageantry. And, to the delight of the nuns, I worked my tail off.

My parents, who had not been religious, followed me into the Church. My mother and Sister Clair Elizabeth Lemer, one of the teachers, became lifelong friends. Sister Clair taught my mother to sew and got her a discount on a Viking sewing machine, which now belongs to my younger sister.

I didn't like Catholic services at first, but learned to love them after I was asked to serve as an altar boy. I worked with Father Ray Ellis, a Lebanese-American priest who would die of a heart attack in his early fifties, when I was in eighth grade. He had the most amazing funeral I have ever seen. Every priest in the diocese and several cardinals were in attendance.

Religion fed my ambition, temporarily causing my dreams to veer away from science. I was obsessed with becoming a bishop. The life of a parish priest wasn't good enough. Later, I saw myself as a Jesuit superior general, or at the very least a Jesuit provincial. For me, religion wasn't about God. It was about playing a leadership role.

After graduating from St. Cecilia, I was admitted to the University of Detroit Jesuit High School, an institution that has consistently been rated among the top prep schools in Michigan.

The U of D High tuition during the 1973/74 school year was $848, which placed it outside my parents' reach. However, Sister Clair came to the rescue. She contacted her brother, the Jesuit provincial responsible for all the Jesuits in Michigan, Ohio, and Indiana. The provincial, in turn, contacted a wealthy alumnus, John Kohl, a U of D High graduate from the class of 1937, who owned a building firm in Traverse City, Michigan. Mr. Kohl agreed to pay my tuition for four years.

My immersion into skepticism was about to begin.

Chapter 5

A Wallet Biopsy

MARTIN SCHMIDT isn't especially concerned about the light-headed, dizzy feeling that sneaks up on him at the office. When you are fifty-eight and working a pressure-cooker job at an express package-delivery company, you learn to expect an off-peak day here and there.

Martin is a broad-shouldered six-footer with a full head of hair and a big, bushy mustache. He played quarterback on his high school football team back in Spartanburg, South Carolina. He married his high school girlfriend, got an associate's degree in business, and moved to Atlanta. Like most people, he grew accustomed to being in robust health, being in control of his life.

Now, weakness starts to descend slowly, like fog. Then, like fog, it lifts. Over the next three days, it returns regularly in waves, at home, at the office. It has logic of its own, lingering longer and longer. Martin starts to fear passing out. Eventually, he does, fading away while starting to dial the number of a difficult client. A coworker finds Martin slumped over his desk, his sleek, black phone emitting frequent, sharp bursts of a siren.

Martin doesn't remember being loaded in an ambulance. He comes to just as the crew wheels him into the emergency room of Piedmont Hospital. Piedmont is one of the more established old hospitals in Atlanta, a place where wealthy and insured people go. By the time the ambulance arrives, Martin is awake and communicating with the EMTs.

The patient's blood pressure is low: 90/50. Listening through a stethoscope, the doctors note that his heart is galloping, 120 beats per minute. Even as Martin's heart pumps harder to keep him alive, the blood is not reaching distant destinations. Extremity pulses are weak. The doctors note a lack of color in Martin's skin.

However, the electrocardiogram, the test that checks the electrical activity of the heart, is normal, except for the heart rate. The lungs are clear, respiratory rate normal, the abdomen soft. When you get a patient like this, you want to rule out the most obvious explanation: heart attack. In this case, there is no evidence of damage to the heart, no sign that a heart attack is in progress.

Martin's blood studies tell more of the story. The hematocrit is low—26 percent. This is a measure of red blood cells in the blood. In an adult male, you expect to see a hematocrit of 42 percent or above. Hemoglobin—a measure of iron-carrying protein in the cells—is similarly low, 8.1 grams per deciliter. Generally, in a healthy adult male, you expect to see 14 g/dl, give or take.

Another blood measurement, the mean corpuscular volume— abbreviated as MCV—points to shrinkage in the average size of his blood cells. You hope to see an MCV of 87 microns. In Martin's case, the blood cells have shriveled to 72. This reading suggests microcytosis, iron deficiency.

Martin has a microcytic anemia, an inadequate amount of blood. Somewhere in his body, he is bleeding. The doctors perform a series of transfusions of packed red blood cells. The objective is to buy time to find the bleed and stop it.

Once myocardial infarction is ruled out, the most common place to lose blood is the gastrointestinal tract. A rectal exam is performed, and a stool sample has the characteristic look of black tar with the classic smell of blood. A smear is placed on a guaiac card (A guaicac is a test of stool looking for blood that might indicate colonic polyps or colon cancer.), and developer solution is added. The paper turns dark blue, indicating the presence of a massive amount of blood.

Martin's gurney is wheeled out to radiology, and he is placed into the oversize, white spinning circle of a computed-tomography scanner. The CT maps out his abdomen in a multitude of image slices. Fortunately, there are no lesions in the liver, but there appears to be a mass in the transverse colon.

By now, thanks to transfusion, Martin's skin has regained more or less its usual color. Tests confirm that the immediate crisis has been managed and there is time to take a detailed look. He is given powerful laxatives in preparation for a colonoscopy. Martin is under sedation, but is vaguely conscious as the doctor slides a scope into his rectum, through the sigmoid colon, past the splenic flexure, to wind through the colon and reach the lesion in the beginning of the transverse colon.

The scope is manipulated past the lesion and eventually to the ileocecal valve, the beginning of the colon. On the way out, several biopsies of the transverse lesion are done though the scope. Two are sent to frozen section to get a quick official answer to what the GI doc already knows.

Martin has a classic presentation of colon cancer.

AFTER anaesthesia clears, Martin and his wife, Rae, are given the diagnosis. Under the circumstances, the news is relatively good. The lesion appears to be localized and could be excised surgically. More often than not, a tumor is more advanced by the time it starts to bleed enough to cause anemia.

Eddie Ghosh, a surgical oncologist, is brought into the case. He sees the patient, reviews the scans and the blood tests. Using a plastic mock-up of the abdomen, he explains Martin's surgery, adding that it needs to be performed sooner rather than later, so that a second cleaning out of the bowel will not be necessary. Sooner, in this case, means late the next day.

The operation report, which would cross my desk later, tells a familiar story: a five-hour procedure, a long abdominal incision, isolation of the section of the colon with the lesion. Then, trouble: the lesion protrudes through the bowel wall.

This is a sign of more advanced disease, pointing to the possibility of spread. Resection of lymph nodes and the involved section of bowel was done without complication. Visual examination of the rest of the large and small bowel, the abdominal wall, and palpation of the liver was normal. Martin's wound was closed, and he was taken to recovery.

Judging by the op report, the surgery was masterful. This is how you do surgery for colon cancer. The surgical oncologist biopsied the abdominal wall and looked for possible lesions on the liver capsule. He even performed an intraoperative ultrasound of the liver to look for evidence of disease.

Things aren't always done this well. In the United States, a general surgeon trained to do hernia repair, hemorrhoid surgery, and appendectomies can perform colon cancer surgery, as can someone who has received extra training as a colorectal surgeon or as a surgical oncologist. The latter two are more likely to do a better job. In most cancers, the quality of the surgery is the most important factor in the ultimate outcome. As one of my favorite surgeons, Charlie Staley, of Emory, likes to say, "You only get one chance to do the surgery right, so choose your surgeon well and pray you have an exceptional surgeon having an exceptionally good day."

THREE days after the surgery, Ghosh introduces Martin to Cameron Wilson, a medical oncologist. The surgeon explains that Martin's cancer went through the bowel wall and spread to six of the twenty-one lymph nodes that were excised during surgery. That's clearly Stage III.

Lymph nodes are like filters, Ghosh explains. The cancer may have been stopped from spreading to the rest of the body by those filters, but a microscopic amount could have gotten past the nodes, which could result in spread to the liver or beyond. Given this, some adjuvant chemotherapy would be necessary to clean up any small amount of cancer in Martin's body.

Hence, Ghosh says, he decided to bring over Wilson. "Dr. Wilson is not just any oncologist," Ghosh says. "Dr. Wilson is *the foremost* oncologist in north Georgia!" It seems the two men know each other well enough for some good-natured teasing.

Ghosh is slight, short, dark-skinned, wearing a tweedy sport coat, but no tie. He has a touch of a British accent and speaks faster than anyone Martin has ever met. Wilson is almost unnaturally tall, reedy. He wears a lawyerly gray suit and a light purple paisley tie. His speech is as unhurried as a day on a North Carolina beach.

The class divide separating Martin from these men is vast. Martin is a middle manager. His job is to please others. He doesn't understand the medical terms (and some nonmedical terms) that have been thrown at him since his ordeal began.

Now, still weak and in pain in his hospital bed, he is getting presentations from men at the top of the medical profession, men who would generally be isolated from him by a cordon of secretaries. Yet, there they are, just three guys talking strategy, like football players huddling before a decisive play.

Wilson's plan is to give Martin a couple of chemotherapy drugs. One has an odd-sounding, short name: 5-FU. The drug will be given to him in single injections. He will also get something called leucovorin, a folatelike vitamin that makes 5-FU work better. The treatment will last for six months.

Also, Martin will get injections under the skin of a drug called erythropoietin, which builds hemoglobin, and a drug called GM-CSF, which builds white blood cells. The first of these drugs will increase the number of Martin's red blood cells, thus keeping him from developing anemia as a side effect of chemotherapy. The second will strengthen his immune system.

Before Martin leaves the hospital, a catheter is placed into a vein under the skin on his chest, to make infusions simpler and less time-consuming.

BEFORE he got sick, Martin, like most Americans, didn't give much thought to big Washington issues such as the cost of health care. Now these problems hit home. Recuperation takes a long time. Martin is weak, he has postoperative pain. Even when times were good, Martin's family lived from paycheck to paycheck, and now with his sick leave exhausted, Martin is too weak to work.

Sick leave runs out the same week Martin shows up for his first appointment with Wilson. Martin still has his job, thank God, and the company still provides insurance, but without a paycheck, copayments on drugs and medical care will soon be ruinous. His deductible is 20 percent on hospital and doctor services, with no coverage for outpatient drugs.

Coveting is not a human foible that afflicts Martin. However, a powerful sense of not-belonging descends on him as he steps through the doors of Wilson's office. While the package-delivery service where Martin works is the picture of clean efficiency, this doctor's office projects an aura of comfort and peaceful contemplation. He walks past a gigantic aquarium and a small rain forest of tropical plants to reach the receptionist, who rises to greet him like a maître d'.

The receptionist, a pretty, young woman who speaks with a down-home drawl, leads Martin and Rae past a taupe, textured wall displaying an impressive collection of photos of Wilson standing next to various prominent Georgia politicians. Sinking into soft velvet chairs beneath the oncologist's wall of respect, Martin and Rae mindlessly fill out the usual forms, feeling out of place and wondering how they will pay for all this.

Before you get to see Wilson, you sit down with his insurance specialist. As Martin and Rae sit uncomfortably in front of her desk, this well-mannered woman in a business suit opens a file and starts explaining how much the treatment regimen will cost. This feels intimidating, like having to agree to a bank loan that you know will strangle you and your family.

Martin will be getting injections of chemotherapy five consecutive days every four weeks for twenty-four weeks. Total estimated costs would be $30,000 to $35,000. His copay, after insurance, would be $6,000 to $7,000. The insurance specialist explains that the office will get reimbursed directly for the 80 percent due from the insurance company, and they want to work out a payment plan for Martin to cover the rest.

Martin admits that he is not sure whether he will be able to return to work and is worried about keeping his insurance while being treated. Here, the lady says something about temporary disability, then something called COBRA, a temporary extension of health insurance after leaving one's job. "I don't know much about these things," she says. "Perhaps you should see a social worker or a financial counselor."

"Perhaps you can recommend one," Rae asks.

"I am afraid I can't."

And that is that.

Wilson's practice serves the elite. Most of his patients are the wives of Atlanta's business leaders getting adjuvant chemotherapy for breast cancer. These women don't work to begin with. Their husbands are the breadwinners, and their insurance is linked to their husbands' jobs.

After that meeting, Martin is ushered into a big room with twelve reclining chairs for the patients. Each has a TV on a swivel arm.

Less comfortable chairs are next to the recliners. These are for people accompanying the patients. The patients are confined to the recliners for chemo administration. Cancer patients have to get used to being sedentary for a long time; some regimens require up to eight hours of sitting. Seven patients, some of them noticeably bald, sit with companions quietly watching TV or trying to sleep as fluids pump slowly from plastic bags into their veins.

A woman introduces herself as "Freda the Chemo Nurse." She starts telling Martin about the chemotherapy and how it will be administered. They will push a needle into the port under his skin and run saltwater through it to hydrate him. Antinausea medicine will go in next, followed by a bolus injection of leucovorin, followed by 5-FU. (Bolus—the word means "ball" in Latin—is fast administration of a drug, a therapeutic blast.) The nurse goes through a litany of side effects, telling Martin what to expect at home in the middle of the night, what drugs she would recommend he take for those side effects. This is a lot of information and a strange world.

Martin takes the chemo without difficulty and feels pretty good afterward. As he and Rae get ready to leave, the nurse hands him a small wad of prescriptions that need to be filled at a pharmacy. For a guy without coverage for prescription meds, this is a concern. He is already trying to figure out how to pay for the chemotherapy at the doctor visits.

That evening, Rae goes to Walgreens and gets the scripts filled. Total cost: $780. She has to put it on the already abused charge card, not even wondering where the money will come from. Martin knows this is not sustainable. Should he just not get care?

Many American cancer patients have to confront the same dilemma. Recently, the American Cancer Society found that one in four Americans undergoing cancer treatment had to put off getting a test or treatment. Among people older than sixty-five, one in five said they had used up all or most of their savings in getting cancer care, and one in seven reported incurring thousands of dollars of medical debt. The survey focused on over a thousand cancer patients and people whose family members have cancer.

Martin is open to the idea of forgoing care, but he has to evaluate it rationally. This requires a talk with Wilson, not just about his finances, but also about his disease. Martin needs his prognosis.

This is urgent: comparing the prognosis with and without chemotherapy is key to the decision to forgo treatment. What is Martin giving up? Alas, Wilson is hard to talk to. During visits, he stops by and says hello as the nurse is readying Martin for 5-FU/leucovorin. He never tarries long enough for Martin to get a word in. Finally, Martin gives up and goes to see the lady in billing.

She is understanding and tells Martin that some people who have had money problems go to Grady. It treats all residents of Fulton and DeKalb Counties regardless of their ability to pay.

Martin considers other alternatives. He has seen commercials for Cancer Treatment Centers of America. They claim to be a group concerned about supporting the patient emotionally. Perhaps they would be more open to discussion than Wilson. He calls them and over the phone learns that treatment there would cost even more than Wilson's. They charge extra for handholding, it seems. He calls other places, and no one is willing to waive the 20 percent deductible.

Finally, Martin has to look at the Grady option. To him, Grady is the county hospital where bums go. It's also where cops go after a shooting or an accident. Burn patients are taken there, too, but outside of emergency care, it's for poor folks. It's not where middle-class people—even middle-class people down on their luck—go.

A thought that Grady is where black people go crosses Martin's mind, too, but he suppresses it, chastising himself for generating a racist, wrong thought. He feels a tinge of shame at it.

MARTIN has difficulty getting an appointment. The administrative part of Grady makes him realize that he is dealing with a government organization akin to the Department of Motor Vehicles.

On the day of his appointment, he and Rae have difficulty parking in the garage next to the hospital. After finding a spot, they get out of the car. The garage is dark, with burnt-out lights. It smells of urine, a big, semi-enclosed toilet for the bums.

They walk past the McDonald's that is carved out of a corner of the garage. They walk past people begging for money. The Grady building itself is imposing, with brown granite running down the façade. At the front entrance, the guards in blue uniforms are conspicuous. Martin and Rae enter a grand but run-down lobby with high ceilings and displays from the history of Atlanta and Grady.

A series of news articles about an Atlanta native, Margaret Mitchell, the author of *Gone with the Wind,* is on display. Mitchell was struck by a car and died at Grady in 1949. Another series of pictures is of a fire that engulfed the Winecoff Hotel on Peachtree Street in downtown Atlanta in 1946. It was one of the worst hotel fires in US history. Another display acknowledges that Grady once ran two nursing schools, one for blacks, one for whites.

Martin and Rae find an elevator bank. One of the doors is gold-colored (it's bronze, actually). A placard says it leads to the Georgia Cancer Center of Excellence. Generally, places that are comfortable with excellence don't call themselves centers of excellence. Has anyone heard of a Princeton University Center of Excellence? Memorial Sloan-Kettering Cancer Center of Excellence?

Installing that elevator might have been the smartest thing I did when I was designing the Grady cancer center. This was a massive renovation of the hospital's ninth and tenth floors, which had been abandoned when the hospital ran out of money during the renovation for the Olympics. Several shafts were left without elevators when the renovation was stopped. I took one of those shafts and bought an elevator. That elevator is dedicated to the cancer center, an express run from the ground floor.

Martin would later tell me that he viewed the elevator as a space vehicle that transported him out of the dreary surroundings of the county hospital to the cancer center, which looked more like a doctor's office in the suburbs.

As the door opens, Martin and Rae enter a room that has bright prints on the walls and clean carpets on the floors. First, Martin has to make arrangements for payment. Grady will bill him for the copays, but will expect him to pay only what he can afford. The hospital writes off the rest. The financial adviser explains that all outpatient prescription drugs will be charged at $2 per prescription. She notes that $2 at Grady even buys drugs that cost $1,000 at regular pharmacies.

Martin and Rae are ushered into an exam room. After a half hour that seems like an eternity, Camille Gray walks in. She is a hematology-oncology fellow. "What is a fellow?" Rae asks. Camille explains that she is a physician who is training to become an oncologist, then asks how she can help. Rae starts to ask why they are seeing a student doctor, but Martin stops her and starts explaining his story to Camille. A student doctor is better than no doctor.

As Martin talks, Camille reads through his records and examines his CT scans. She asks a few questions about the chemo that he has received, verifying the schedule, trying to verify the drugs. Martin doesn't know the names of all the meds, but he does remember 5-FU.

Camille examines him, to make sure the physical findings are consistent with the history. He has a little mild mucositis, rawness in the mouth, a result of chemotherapy. His belly scar is healing well. No lymph nodes are palpable in the neck and upper clavicle area. The liver and spleen are not palpable, the belly is soft, and there are no masses. His labs drawn a week earlier are indicative of chemotherapy a few days before.

Our fellows are taught to verify everything in a patient's story for consistency with the record and the exam. Occasionally, we get people who tell compelling stories that fail to check out. They come to us because they want attention or, worse, in hopes of scoring some "good drugs," narcotics for recreational use or street commerce.

Around the corner from Grady, a single Vicodin tablet goes for $20.

CAMILLE leaves the room and prepares to "present the case." Presenting the case is a century-old medical tradition. Other fellows and students, one other attending who is not busy, and some nurses, nurse's aides, a social worker, and some patient navigators gather in the multipurpose room in the former white section of the tenth floor to hear Camille discuss Martin's case.

All young physicians and even some of us middle-aged ones are called on to present. The order of information in the presentation is the same today as it was more than a century ago. The only change is the modern addition of results of lab tests and imaging studies.

Camille addresses the presentation to me, the attending in charge of the clinic that day: "Mr. Schmidt is a fifty-eight-year-old white male with a two-month history of Stage IIIB adenocarcinoma of the colon. He was diagnosed initially at Piedmont Hospital, after presenting with loss of consciousness due to anemia. He was found to have a colon cancer in the transverse colon."

I am of the school that believes that medical education need not be boring. "Let me guess. Mr. Schmidt's wallet biopsy turned up negative," I throw in.

Camille smiles. Of course it's the wallet biopsy, the means test revealing inability to pay. Can there be any other explanation for a guy who gets initial care at a rich-people hospital to turn up here at Grady?

She proceeds with clinical details: "CT of the liver is negative. It was resected in a good operation, and he recovered well. He began chemotherapy with bolus 5-FU and leucovorin and now comes to Grady because he cannot afford the chemotherapy."

"What do 5-FU and Otis Brawley have in-common?" I ask.

"Hmm . . ." Camille rolls her eyes. "You are also a thymidylate synthase inhibitor?"

Good, she knows the mechanism of action of 5-FU. Camille tilts her head to the right and looks at me with expectation of some absurdity.

"Age," I say. "Five-FU was first used in chemotherapy in 1959; Otis Brawley was born in 1959. We've been doing the same bullshit for fifty years."

I mean this, at least half of it: 5-FU is a marginally effective drug. For a long time, we didn't even know whether it increased the patients' survival. Yet, for a couple of generations, gastrointestinal oncologists prescribed it to desperate patients. Since there was nothing else around, it was the standard of care. Leucovorin is a folinic acid. It's believed to work synergistically with 5-FU.

Camille smiles at the joke and proceeds to a suggested treatment plan. "As Dr. Brawley noted, 5-FU/leucovorin is an obsolete regimen for a healthy man with the status postsurgery for Stage III disease."

I start out at the presentation knowing nothing about the case, like a priest sitting in a confessional. Camille's presentation has intrigued me, and I begin thumbing through the papers in front of me. I glance at the patient data and the surgery report. "Does this gentleman stand to benefit from chemotherapy?" I ask, continuing to look through the loose pages in front of me.

Of course Camille knows the answer, but I want be sure that she is able to recite these facts with poise at a patient's bedside.

"The literature indicates that he does," Camille says—correctly.

A patient with Stage III colon cancer has a 50 percent to 60 percent chance of its recurring, she continues. She cites randomized trials done in the 1980s that 5-FU–based therapy could lower the chance of death by about 30 percent. This reduction in relative risk translated into a 10 percent boost in five-year survival.

"Is there any controversy over this?" I ask.

"No," says Camille, citing a 1990 consensus conference that recommended that all Stage III patients whose disease had been fully removed surgically and who are medically fit to withstand chemotherapy should be treated with 5-FU.

"So, should we also treat this gentleman with 5-FU?" I throw in. It's another trick question.

"No," says Camille. "Five-FU as a single agent or 5-FU with a modulator like leucovorin would have been appropriate in 1990, but not today. I believe we should consider treating this gentleman with FOLFOX."

Correct. FOLFOX is a combination regimen that includes the newer drug oxaliplatin in addition to 5-FU/leucovorin. Oxali is a platinum drug that has been used extensively in colorectal cancer. Platinum drugs are made of hydrogen and carbon molecules around one molecule of platinum. The first platinum drug was Cis-Platinum, which is commonly used to treat lung cancer and is part of the curative regimen for testicular cancer. Camille quotes a trial called the Multicenter International Study of Oxaliplatin, 5-Fluorouracil, and Leucovorin in the Adjuvant Treatment of Colon Cancer as evidence to support her assertion. This trial—its name is abbreviated as MOSAIC—redefined the way we treat colon cancer.

MOSAIC showed a five-year disease-free survival rate of 73 percent in the FOLFOX arm and 67 percent in the 5-FU-leucovorin arm. This result was statistically significant, meaning that it was unlikely to be a fluke—FOLFOX was a better treatment.

The increased survival rate with FOLFOX comes at a cost of peripheral neuropathy, which in 12 percent of cases becomes severe. This is no small problem. A patient receiving this drug may have difficulty buttoning his or her clothes. But the improvement in outcomes is significant enough to become the standard of care.

"When would 5-FU/leucovorin only—without oxali—be appropriate?" I ask, looking for the name of the guy who treated Martin.

"I would consider it for a little old lady with Stage III colon cancer, who was otherwise healthy and appeared to have a less than ten-year life expectancy," Camille says.

The oxaliplatin in FOLFOX might be too harsh for an older patient, but a fifty-eight-year-old otherwise healthy guy can tolerate it, and studies say his risk of relapse would go down a bit. Camille is right. Five-year survival with FOLFOX is better than 65 percent. Martin's chances of survival are far worse—and not quantifiable—with lousy treatment. Any patient deserves every effort to do the treatment right.

Camille continues, "Even if I were giving 5-FU/leucovorin alone, I would not give bolus, which is what this patient was getting. I would give it by continuous infusion."

"Why?" I ask.

Camille talks about the clinical studies that have shown that infusional 5-FU has different side effects from a bolus. A bolus is the fast way to give 5-FU, and that's not a good thing. Literature shows that slow methods of administration—an infusion pump that dispenses the drug over twenty-four hours or so—is not as toxic.

Before newer drugs came along, GI oncologists busied themselves trying to define the best way to give 5-FU. (This was kind of sad. There were no other drugs, nothing else to study.)

The regimen Wilson was giving Martin, called the Mayo Clinic Regimen, had been surpassed as the preferred regimen by the Roswell Park Regimen, Camille says. It's less toxic. It's a once-weekly 5-FU/leucovorin given for four eight-week courses. She then says that she likes another method, the de Gramont Regimen, even more. In this regimen, 5-FU is given by long-term continuous infusion.

"Does everyone here remember *Forrest Gump*?" I say. I can't help it. It's one of my favorite movies, and many things in life—at least my life—remind me of it. "I think of what Forrest Gump says of the various ways to serve shrimp," I continue through the giggles. "You can give 5-FU by IV bolus, you can give it by twenty-four-hour infusion, you can give it by five-day infusion, you can give it by seven-day infusion, you can give it with leucovorin, you can give it in oral form, which is toxic and expensive as shit. It just goes on and on. I mean, really, why would anyone give 5-FU/leucovorin to a patient who can tolerate something better? The thought of it pisses me off."

"Beats me," says Camille. "Maybe the physician in question hasn't kept up with the literature."

"He'd have to be brain-dead to have missed the literature," I offer. "What's his name anyway?" I had seen the name by now, but it's important to let the name come out. Bad docs tend to resurface, and it's important to be prepared.

"That would be Dr. Cameron Wilson," she says, and I decide not to press further. Wilson was, in effect, depriving Martin of a chance of a better outcome, perhaps even a cure. I wanted to look at the charts to see for myself what might have been going through Wilson's mind.

After everyone leaves, I stay on, continuing to thumb through the chart, interrogating it, trying to grasp its deeper meaning. What I see frightens me.

If you are poor, black, and uninsured like Edna, you get no care until it's too late. This is no surprise to anyone. But if you are rich, white, and insured, you face another deadly menace, a Dr. Wilson, a socially prominent physician who is just plain bad. As a patient, you would see his social prominence—he might even belong to your country club—but you would have no way to see his inadequacy as a physician.

Even the surgeon who did a competent resection recommended this doctor to Martin. If you can't trust a recommendation of your surgeon, what can you trust?

Reviewing the chart, I am unable to understand why Wilson agreed to take on Martin. Colon cancer isn't even his area of specialization. Oncologists, like all doctors, get better at something if they do it all the time. Wilson did a lot of adjuvant therapy for breast cancer, and with the exception of his overuse of supportive-care drugs, he did it reasonably well. For

him, adjuvant chemo for breast cancer was relatively easy, like following a recipe from a cookbook. You only have to be an adequate doctor
to do this well. Providing adjuvant therapy for breast cancer is a great
place to be mediocre: no clinical judgments need be made, and the money
is good.

Did Wilson want to diversify? Were his sales lagging? Did he think
Martin's insurance was too good to pass up? I don't know. What I do
know is that a doctor like him would have been weeded out at Grady. At
Grady, we have standards for treatment of commonly seen diseases. These
standards take into account the national and international treatment
guidelines and receive input from Emory's disease-specific experts. The
doctors at Emory who only treat GI cancer also rotate through Grady and
are charged with verifying that our standard of care for colon cancer is
appropriate.

We look over each other's shoulder to see how we are treating patients.
This is an added degree of quality control that you do not see in private
practice and sometimes not even in an academic practice. The system at
Grady does allow for varying from the standard of care, but we have to
discuss it with peers and with our patients. We have to have a valid reason
for deviation. This means solid medical literature, not the pleadings of a
drug rep, even if she offers a free meal and tickets to the Falcons-Saints
game.

Camille had only twenty-five minutes to make her presentation, and
there was a lot to talk about. I deliberately focused on the standard of
care for Martin's disease. Now, as I stare at the papers, I look at Wilson's
use of a drug that builds red blood cells and another drug that builds
white blood cells. These are expensive drugs that the patient likely didn't
need. I see no indication that Martin was anemic or that his white blood
cells were down low enough to justify a pharmacological intervention.

At Grady, we use white-blood-cell-building drugs only on folks who
have a bout of fever due to low white cell count. Red-blood-cell-building
drugs are used only when a patient develops symptoms of anemia while
getting chemotherapy. At the time of Martin's treatment, supportive-
care drugs were a standard booster for an oncologist's bottom line. Overtreatment with these drugs was common and was driven by market

forces. Drug manufacturers gave volume discounts to private practices. The more doctors used, the greater their profits. As they boosted the cost of care, the patient's copayments rose as well.

Many of Wilson's treatment decisions seem mystifying even if you accept the notion that his goal was to maximize profits. The treatment he chose for Martin isn't known to justify the use of supportive medications. Had he wanted to justify the use of these drugs, he could have sold Martin on FOLFOX. This would have allowed him to collect the profit from oxaliplatin, which is far more expensive than 5-FU/leucovorin. Moreover, oxaliplatin's more severe side effects might have made Martin sick enough to justify giving him red-and white-blood-cell-building drugs.

Wilson was not interested enough in either maximizing his profits or in giving the patient appropriate care. He simply threw treatments at Martin without thinking, collecting the money that came his way. Never mind that the treatments were wrong and perhaps damaging. He simply didn't care. He seemed to be motivated by a puzzling combination of laziness and greed.

I have some tolerance for below-average or average doctors who know their limits and stay within them. Doctors who don't know the limits of their knowledge are another matter. Doctors who don't know what they don't know—and don't care—are dangerous.

I meet Martin in person a week later. We have a lot to discuss, and I struggle to decide how much I should tell him.

Should I tell him that his previous doctor was a dangerous ignoramus? Would he benefit from this knowledge?

I tell residents and fellows to avoid criticizing other doctors in similar situations. If I tell Martin the things he deserves to know, I risk being hauled into court for slander by Wilson. Alternatively, if Martin decides to sue his former physician, I could get hauled into court as an expert witness.

No doctor can clean up the profession all by himself.

I limit myself to telling Martin that I would have offered him a different chemo regimen: "I—and the medical literature—have a preference for a regimen that contains a drug called oxaliplatin." I am careful to explain how the medical staff agreed that chemotherapy was called for. I explain that there is more than one way to skin a cat, and that there is more than one way to treat colon cancer. I give him a choice of chemotherapy options, explaining the pros and cons. I explain what we know, what we do not know, and what we believe about his disease and its treatment. FOLFOX increases the chances of a cure, but this comes at a cost of peripheral neuropathy and possible leukemia down the road. My policy is to explain the entire picture—including outcomes, side effects, and inconvenience to lifestyle—to the patient and let him decide on therapy.

When patients say, "What should I do, Doc?" you try to work it out with them.

Martin mentions his desire to return to work while getting chemotherapy and notes that this is important to his family's financial health. I tell him that I understand, and I do. My parents lived from paycheck to paycheck throughout my childhood. I want Martin to understand that my compassion is genuine. It is, too. I don't want to fake it. I can't.

As I discuss treatment strategies with Martin, I don't want my skin color to distract him. Race evokes different responses from different people in different settings, and I don't want it to get in the way. I can't forget for an instant that I am a black guy dealing with a white guy in the South.

I am a black guy in authority, and for the sake of my patients I can't afford to trip over land mines. It's not about me. The stakes are high for Martin: the things I say, things I do, will shape our relationship and with it the rest of Martin's life. I don't know whether keeping this at the forefront of my mind makes me a better doctor, but it does keep me sensitive to the importance of the doctor-patient relationship.

Eventually, we decide to try FOLFOX, even though I take care to tell him that I have no data on someone treated with one regimen and switched to another.

Next, we turn to logistics. I tell him that I would be the attending physician responsible for his care. Camille would be his fellow, doing day-to-day care for only six months. After that, Camille would move on, and Martin would have to adjust to other fellows.

Passing through the clinic over the next year I develop a good relationship with Martin and Rae. He becomes comfortable enough with me to discuss his concerns about coming to Grady and his shame in thinking this is where black people get care. I tell him about my fears of white people. We laugh.

Martin continues to get follow-up surveillance at Grady, and four years after treatment ended he is disease-free.

A negative wallet biopsy may have saved his life.

RECENTLY, I heard about a pediatric orthopedic surgeon's disastrous job interview with a large practice group in the Northeast.

"We have a strict rule here," one of the practice leaders told him. "We eat what we kill."

Behind the curtain, when no patient was within earshot, this revolting metaphor told the interviewee that members at that practice are responsible for bringing in business, and their ability to attract patients determines their pay.

You can't help getting crass in medicine. Training starts early. The stuff you hear—and the stuff you say—as a resident, particularly during ER rotation, is unacceptable in any civilized setting. We doctors ultimately live in two worlds that require two forms of self-expression. In one world, we speak openly to our colleagues, without niceties. In the other setting—when patients are around—most of us try to behave, at least to the best of our ability.

Surgeons tend to be more resilient than other docs, and the surgeon who told me this story isn't a meek soul. But the hunting metaphor offended him deeply. Having just returned from earthquake-stricken Haiti, where he performed gruesome amputations of the limbs of children who had been pulled out of rubble, he was in no mood for crass talk that debased human life. In no way could he force himself to join a practice where it's okay to talk about patients as things that are killed and eaten.

Every time I hear a story like this, I praise the gods for going easy on me. I work for a big public charity and I practice at a big public hospital.

I chose this life, gravitating toward research and, to the extent possible, shielding myself from the perverse incentives that entice my colleagues to do harm. I have no overhead to cover, no sales targets, no worries about Medicare reimbursement policies and insurers who take too long to pay.

Would I be a very different doc if I were out there in private practice? Would I preserve the moral principles to refer out the patients whose diseases I don't understand well enough to treat? Would I be willing to forgo the five- or six-figure revenues that treating such a patient could bring to my practice? So what if I give him some bullshit? So what if I don't know what I am doing?

Revenues, after all, aren't smeared with blood. They are numbers on a page. They aren't dependent on whether I help my patients or harm them. And if I screw up, is there a reason to believe that anyone would be the wiser?

PART II

Failure Is the System

Chapter 6

Red Juice

IN 1995, Lilla Romeo was living a happy life as an American professional in Europe. Lilla's husband, Anthony, was an executive for Unilever, a global food and personal-care-products company, in London, and she was selling Mercedes cars in Kent. They were raising three children.

When Lilla was first diagnosed with breast cancer, it seemed to be only a minor setback. The disease was caught early—in Stage I—and surgery followed by radiation had a good shot at curing her. Statistically, the chances were three to one that the problem would simply go away after treatment; with cancer, you don't ask for better odds.

Lilla was in the unlucky 25 percent. Five years after the initial diagnosis, when the family was back in New York, a routine scan showed that the disease had returned. The prognosis turned grim. The cancer was incurable, and the goal of treatment was to delay the inevitable. Lilla started nonstop chemotherapy.

When we talk on the phone in 2010, Lilla has been on chemo for nearly ten years with just one eight-month break. (Doctors inventively call such interludes "chemo holidays.") Lilla is an intensely analytical person. Her phrases are chiseled to the point of fragility. She takes time to think, then pauses to let her words sink in deep and do their work.

She remembers the day in 2003 when an oncology nurse at New York University Medical Center asked if she was feeling tired. Lilla gave the question a little thought. Of course, she was a bit worn down. What else would you expect to hear from someone going into year four of nonstop chemo? She answered affirmatively.

"That would be because your hemoglobin is just under ten," the nurse explained. Lilla was on the borderline of developing anemia, a common side effect of the cancer drugs. The nurse explained that in the old days, a patient like Lilla would get a blood transfusion. This cumbersome procedure involves tubes and hours in the doctor's office. Worse, transfusions carry the risk of HIV and other blood-borne infections. By 2003, thanks to better blood-screening technology, that risk had been lowered, but there was still a risk.

Now, the nurse said, almost the same results could be attained with a single shot of a hormone that helps the body produce hemoglobin. The nurse made it seem simple, safe, clean. The red blood cells Lilla needed would be made by her own body.

Lilla knew something about cancer-fatigue drugs. In 2003, everyone with cancer—and some without—did. That's because Johnson & Johnson, the gigantic pharmaceutical company, was bombarding the airwaves with ads for its hemoglobin-producing drug Procrit. Procrit ads depicted heartwarming scenes in which cancer patients spoke of the drug's miraculous ability to restore the "strength for living" that had been drained by cancer chemotherapy.

In one ad, an owner of a New England bed-and-breakfast thanks Procrit for giving him the strength to confront the busy season. In another, an elderly African American woman says proudly that Procrit had given her the strength to make an omelet. A grandfather throws a giggling grandson up in the air, and an elderly white woman has regained the strength to return to running her flower shop. "More red blood cells can mean more strength," the ad says. Cancer is losing its power to rob people of normal life. The effects of cancer treatment have become easier to tolerate.

Lilla is a born skeptic, and after a career in sales she understands the liberties people take in marketing. Yet, as she sits in the treatment room in 2003, Lilla sees no reason to believe that her situation calls for hard-nosed analysis. How could there possibly be a controversy? Surely the Food and Drug Administration had approved Procrit for making cancer patients feel stonger. Would the agency approve a drug that would harm her? And surely the FDA was overseeing those televised ads. Isn't that part of what that agency does?

She had no idea that her infusion chair was the front-row seat for observing a spectacular, indeed, cataclysmic, failure in medicine. Pharmaceutical companies were promoting an untested therapy that was purported to make patients feel better and stronger when, in fact, it caused strokes and heart attacks and in some cases made tumors grow. My colleagues didn't object. The vast majority of physicians treating cancer were prescribing these drugs and benefiting handsomely from doing so. Prescribing these drugs created enough of a financial bonanza for doctors that many of them turned off their professional skepticism.

Cancer patients and their doctors routinely accept horrific risks as they inject drugs intended to cure cancer or slow down its process. Alas, hemoglobin-building drugs did nothing of the sort. They treated anemia, and, according to claims made in advertising, made patients feel better.

Until the FDA finally clamped down, these drugs became the single largest category of agents used in oncology.

You can't scrutinize everything, even if you are a skeptic by nature. When you are a patient confronting a devastating disease you know next to nothing about, and decisions have to be made in a hurry, you end up having to trust somebody.

Certainly, no patient can be expected to take the weeks or months that would be required to conduct a critical examination of the criteria a federal agency used when it approved a particular therapy.

Lilla delegated decisions to the doctors and nurses at the cancer center where she was receiving treatment. She was sure the doctors wouldn't recommend a drug that would be inappropriate for a breast-cancer patient. Lilla had enough problems; her anemia, which she now believed was causing fatigue, didn't need to be one of them.

She remembers feeling a little better after getting a shot.

Those were paradoxical years for hemoglobin-building drugs. Sales of this category of drugs grew explosively, making them the largest-selling class of drugs used in oncology, with 2006 gross sales of $4.85 billion in the United States alone. That year, worldwide sales were $10 billion.

At the same time, evidence of harm—including strokes, heart attacks, and something the FDA called "tumor promotion"—accumulated with alarming consistency. *Tumor promotion* is an Orwellian term. It stands for the drug's ability to make tumors *grow*.

Neither Lilla nor millions of other cancer patients—particularly those with breast and head-and-neck cancer—had any reason to suspect that the drugs they received for counteracting anemia were doing real, measurable harm.

Lilla was simply taking the treatment her medical team suggested would ease her situation.

IN 2003—the year Lilla first received Procrit—my skepticism about that drug was in part instinctive and in part based on evidence. I simply was not convinced that these drugs were worth the potential risks, and J&J's aggressive advertising campaign only increased my skepticism. Direct-to-consumer ads during the Super Bowl and the evening news makes my prescription pad retreat deeper into my pocket. As a physician, I need to see the data, not advertising. Ideally, I need to see a comparison of the results of multiple patients receiving Treatment A and an equal number of patients receiving Treatment B or placebo. That's the gold standard in the hierarchy of evidence.

When pressed, I can make do with trials that don't have a comparator arm (by which I mean trials that don't have patients that are receiving Treatment B). They are less reliable, but better than nothing. The opinions of my esteemed colleagues don't hold much water with me because we doctors are routinely proven wrong. The anecdote—the experience of a single patient—is less valuable still.

Direct-to-consumer ads are the least valuable way of describing the true value of a treatment. Television spots don't even pretend to reflect the experiences of real people. They are scripted and staged to convince cancer patients to pressure their doctors to prescibe drugs that the patients and their insurers will pay for.

I saw no point in asking my patients whether they were feeling fatigued. It's the sort of question that suggests—indeed predetermines—an affirmative answer. You ask twenty-five healthy people if they are tired, and the majority will say yes. And so J&J's Super Bowl advertising was selling a problem as much as a solution. In fact, the company manufactured a medical condition: cancer fatigue.

What cancer patient isn't going to report feeling fatigued? Their bodies are being undermined by both the disease and interventions seeking to control it.

Though I didn't specifically follow all the literature on anemia drugs, I did read the thirty-plus-page insert, a document that summarizes clinical data and other materials on drugs approved by the FDA. (Few doctors read the entire label before prescribing a drug. I do.) In 2003, the data in the Procrit label did nothing to calm my misgivings.

I don't claim to be uncommonly insightful, but I am a good student, and I am consistent in interpretating evidence. It's always about the balance of what I know, what I don't know, and what I believe.

The man who taught me the most about evaluation of evidence, Father Richard Polakowski, had never been to medical school. He taught eleventh-grade English at the University of Detroit Jesuit High School. Father Polakowski had a maxim that no student who took his class could miss: "Say what you know, what you don't know, and what you believe—and label it accordingly."

When I took his class in 1975, Polo (Father Polakowski's nickname) was about fifty. A slight man, he retained a childish, lisping manner of pronunciation. Polo taught a heavyweight curriculum: Chaucer, Shakespeare, Elie Wiesel, Chinua Achebe, Yasunari Kawabata, Isaac Bashevis Singer, Graham Greene, Richard Wright.

By year's end, all of us became experts in applying Polo's maxim to literary criticism. Use your intellect, gentlemen. Start with knowledge, find its boundary. Do not stop! Save room for belief, but examine it fearlessly, for genuine examination knows no limitation.

Polo concluded his multicultural blitz with *A Portrait of the Artist as a Young Man,* James Joyce's reflection on his Jesuit education. "Some people read about it, gentlemen," Polo said. "You are *living* it." You could see how proud he was to teach a criticism of the institution he was a part of, the institution he loved. It takes a special combination of humility and pride to invite a group of would-be young artists—or at least young contrarians—to tear apart their teacher, their school, the religious order that runs it, and, if they so choose, God Himself.

Examination thus practiced can be deeply unsettling. A priori, you have to accept the consequences of acting on your conclusions, whether these include a crisis of faith, a bleeding ulcer, an excommunication, or an insurrection.

Polo's maxim quickly turned into my favorite device for exploring the universe. Over the years, I've applied it to everything I do, from epidemiology to the design of clinical trials to the discussion of treatment options with my patients. Much of what we do in oncology requires balancing benefits against harm. Harm can include conventional metrics such as blood clots, but also cost to the patient and society. Sometimes we treat one hundred people to benefit ten. All one hundred will be subjected to harm, and ninety people will pay the price for the lucky ten. Patients need to be informed about uncertainty in order to decide to roll the dice or sit out the game. If you truly respect the patients you treat, you will not obscure the line where your knowledge stops and your opinion begins. It's the only decent thing to do.

I consider myself religious, but not overly religious. Polo convinced me that God expects us to work for social justice, and the best way to serve Him is through caring for others. Some people praise God by going to church on Sunday. I seek to do the same daily by helping those in distress—and by telling the truth.

FROM the outset, the things I knew and the things I didn't know about Procrit—and another anemia drug, Aranesp—made me believe that I was observing a systemic failure in medicine.

The evidence that led to Procrit's approval had been remarkably—spectacularly—unconvincing. The FDA approved the drug for the treatment of anemia in cancer patients in 1993, ten years before it was offered to Lilla. The approval was based on data pooled from six remarkably small studies that altogether enrolled a total of only 131 patients. Generally, the FDA doesn't approve drugs based on pooled studies, which are also called meta-analyses. This is because a meta-analysis can be only as good as the studies it pools. In the case of Procrit, the agency rolled the dice. The nation's blood banks were threatened by the AIDS epidemic, and the prospect of finding a hormone that would induce the body to produce its own hemoglobin was enticing.

Yet, even if the Procrit data *had* come from a single study, the total number of patients would have been unconvincing. That's because the patients in these studies had a variety of tumors, which presented another problem. There was no way to measure how Procrit behaved in this mixed bag of diagnoses. Would its impact on a patient with early-stage breast cancer differ from its impact on advanced colon cancer?

The six minuscule trials from which the data were pooled had not asked the questions I needed answered before I would reach for a prescription pad. The studies asked only whether Procrit had the ability to prevent blood transfusions. (Procrit accomplished this well enough to get on the market.) However, before I would be convinced to start giving this drug to my patients, I needed to know about Procrit's toxicity as well as its impact on survival, or at least on the tempo of cancer's progression. Did people who received Procrit face a higher risk of blood clots? Did their underlying cancer recur? Did they die sooner? Was their anemia corrected? Did the answers to these questions differ from cancer to cancer? These questions were unanswered.

Reading Procrit's label critically, I saw that not a shred of data said anything about either "fatigue" or its opposite, "strength." Those words—which were central to the direct-to-consumer ads—were simply not on the label. Yes, anemia is associated with fatigue, but would correction of anemia—pushing the hemoglobin levels into a higher range—alleviate fatigue? There was no way to know, certainly not based on data. The claims of giving patients "strength for living" were completely, blatantly unsupported. I couldn't understand why the FDA had not pulled the plug on the J&J ads. (The answers would emerge later, when a congressional investigation would unearth evidence that FDA scientists attempted to stop those ads. However, pro-industry attorneys appointed by the Bush administration to run the agency's top legal office blocked the scientists' efforts.)

The manner in which many of my colleagues prescribed these drugs made me increasingly uneasy. The problem I saw was overtreatment, and overtreatment equals harm.

If you accepted that Procrit was equivalent to a blood transfusion (which we had no evidence for), it would make sense to use it in a way that mirrors the use of blood transfusions. Normally, we transfuse patients who are suffering from significant anemia. No blood bank will release blood for a patient whose hemoglobin is above 8.5 g/dl. However, an ever-increasing number of my colleagues considered it justifiable to give Procrit to patients whose red blood cells were at much higher levels. Lilla got it at 10 g/dl. Generally, doctors thought it was reasonable to give the drug to patients whose hemoglobin was sliding below 12 g/dl. Some didn't bother to check what the patent's hemoglobin was and erred on the side of giving Procrit every time they gave chemo. This was spectacularly efficacious for the doctor's wallet, but harmful to the patients and the health-care system.

Furthermore, doctors routinely prescribed the drugs for uses in which it had not been studied—such as anemia caused by cancer itself, as opposed to anemia caused by chemotherapy. I know of a case where a patient was sent to hospice with a supply of syringes filled with these drugs.

At the time Lilla got her first injection of Procrit, J&J and a competitor, Amgen Inc., were pursuing studies aimed at pushing the cancer patients' hemoglobin to "near-normal range," which they defined as 14 g/dl and above. These were exceedingly puzzling clinical trials, in part because no one can say with certainty what the normal level of hemoglobin should be.

Fatigue is in the eye of the beholder. It's hard to measure it objectively, and asking people whether they are feeling tired will not do the trick. I know that many of my patients are not aware that their hemoglobin is at 8 g/dl. Healthy pregnant women do extremely well at 7.5 g/dl. A Denver resident can have a hemoglobin level a full point above that of her cousin in Wichita, Kansas. This happens because the air in the Mile High City contains less oxygen than the air on the Great Plains. Would this justify putting Procrit in Wichita's water supply?

No scientific study has shown that a particular level of hemoglobin is important. As a clinician, you have to consider these levels based on the patient's characteristics. A patient with coronary artery disease usually experiences a shortness of breath as she walks up a flight of stairs when her hemoglobin drops to 8.5 g/dl. However, for a fifty-year-old woman in good shape, the 8.5 g/dl level is no problem unless she decides to run a mile or two.

Hemoglobin's importance isn't lost on athletes, which is why these same hemoglobin-building drugs are often used as an illegal doping agent. We need oxygen to perform better. We also know that our bodies adjust to variations in oxygen levels. This is why football teams often go to Denver a couple of days before playing there. Practicing at that altitude for three or four days helps players adjust (though it takes two weeks or so to become completely acclimated).

But Lilla wasn't competing in the Tour de France or playing football in Denver. No data suggested that her self-reported "tiredness" had any clinical significance or that increasing her hemoglobin level would make her feel better. Since nothing was known about the potential for improvement, there was no way to weigh it against potential costs, which include side effects and the cost of treatment.

No matter how I looked at it, I couldn't justify prescribing these drugs to a patient like Lilla, who was not presenting with any symptoms of anemia and was doing reasonably well.

Why was she prompted to say that she was "fatigued" only to be given a drug that was not proven to have the ability to correct fatigue? Why were these doctors treating a number on a chart instead of treating Lilla Romeo?

LILLA believed she received Procrit roughly four times a year. Each time, she needed at least two shots to get her hemoglobin to 12 g/dl.

In 2004, she was told that the hospital had switched from Procrit to another drug, Aranesp, which supposedly had a longer-lasting effect and therefore required fewer shots. Lilla could tell the difference between the two drugs. Aranesp caused a burning sensation under her skin at the injection site.

"I remember saying that it stings, and I would much prefer Procrit," Lilla recalled. However, she was told that Procrit was no longer available, as the hospital had shifted to the Amgen drug.

As a marketing expert, Lilla would have been interested in the nasty warfare between J&J, the company that sold Procrit, and Amgen, the company that sold Aranesp. She might have been even more interested in examining the intricate financial incentives Amgen had created to induce oncologists to prescribe more Aranesp.

In oncology, it's rare to find a drug that is used to treat a variety of tumors. Since areas of cancer treatment are becoming increasingly specialized, it's unlikely that we will see another Taxol, a drug used for lung, ovarian, breast, and head-and-neck cancer, as well as advanced Kaposi's sarcoma. It's also unlikely that we will see many drugs that can be used to treat all patients with a particular tumor, such as all breast cancers, all colon cancers, or all lung cancer. Many of today's drugs are developed to treat minuscule numbers of patients, and as development efforts become more focused—say, on diseases associated with particular genetic characteristics—it will be common to see drugs that may help a thousand or two thousand new patients a year.

Procrit and Aranesp bucked that trend. As supportive-care drugs, they could be used in patients undergoing chemotherapy for any solid tumor. You could give it to every patient, unless the patient had blood cancer.

Doctors don't have to prescribe drugs based strictly for uses listed on the FDA label. They prescribed these drugs "off label," too, giving them to patients with blood cancers and patients whose anemia was attributed to cancer itself, as opposed to chemotherapy.

Doctors could also prescribe these drugs for anemia associated with kidney disease, AIDS, and surgery. The market was gigantic.

The treatment of anemia was anyone's dream franchise, the sort of thing people don't give up voluntarily.

YOU can entice or bully doctors into a consensus. You can invent a medical condition called cancer fatigue, stage skits, and play them during the Super Bowl to convince patients that a simple prescription can make their tiredness go away. You can do all this, but sooner or later, nature will look you in the eye and, after making sure that you are paying attention, give you the middle finger.

Soon after hemoglobin-building drugs were approved, a German radiation therapist named Michael Henke decided to test one of the fundamental tenets of his subspecialty: that patients with higher hemoglobin levels have better responses to radiation therapy. Though this assumption was untested, it had made its way into textbooks.

Henke believed in the connection between hemoglobin and response to radiation. His goal in trying to officially prove it was to demonstrate that increasing a patient's hemoglobin with a Procrit-like drug would bring about better outcomes. He was such a true believer that the Swiss drug company Roche gave him access to its own hemoglobin-boosting drug and research funding for a 351-patient study, which he started in 1997. Roche was happy to help out. A positive study would likely have led to regulatory approvals and expansion of what was already a lucrative franchise.

The study's results didn't come out the way Henke expected.

He was shocked.

"I was a strong believer, but sometimes you see different things," he told a reporter in 2003, after his results were published. The study showed that patients who received the hemoglobin-building drug didn't live as long as those on placebo. Also, the disease progressed more rapidly in patients receiving the drug.

Henke concluded that he had encountered a biological phenomenon: the drug seemed to be encouraging tumors to grow.

When a reporter called an Amgen source to discuss Henke's findings, the source said that Henke was a gadfly who didn't understand clinical research, a well-meaning boob.

I didn't think Henke was a boob. His findings reinforced my concerns that anemia-building drugs were overused. Several of my academic colleagues agreed with me. After publication of Henke's results, doctors at Emory and at the University of Texas MD Anderson Cancer Center in Houston stopped prescribing these agents to patients with treatable head-and-neck cancer. However, doctors in private practice or at private hospitals and cancer centers continued to prescribe these drugs. Sales figures indicate that most docs and most hospitals didn't dwell on Henke's important findings and, for the most part, either didn't pay attention or didn't care.

In August 2003, researchers had to stop another study, the Breast Cancer Erythropoietin Survival Trial, abbreviated as BEST. In that trial, more women died on Proctit than on the control arm. This result, obtained from that massive 939-patient study, was more relevant to Lilla's case. In this study, patients received Procrit when their hemoglobin level dropped below 13 g/dl. In both the Henke trial and BEST, the survival curve showed an increased risk of death from cancer, which suggested something you don't want to see in patients you are treating for cancer: tumor growth.

This finding was so shocking that the principal investigator of the BEST study, incredibly, cautioned doctors against drawing far-reaching conclusions.

"It is extremely unfortunate that the problems in design, conduct, and post-trial analysis have complicated the interpretation of this study," the principal investigator, Brian Leyland-Jones, then of McGill University in Montreal, wrote in *The Lancet Oncology* in August 2003. "Given the number of design issues uncovered in the post hoc analyses, the results cannot be considered conclusive."

Usually, clinical researchers live and die by their data. Here, the data were so much at odds with medical practice and prevailing beliefs that Leyland-Jones was urging his colleagues to disregard the evidence and go by his opinion instead. Never before had I seen such guidance in medical literature.

After BEST, people I respect in breast cancer became cautious about Procrit and Aranesp. On the pharmaceutical end of things, far from disregarding Leyland-Jones's findings, J&J decided to stop all studies where the treatment goal was to push hemoglobin into the so-called normal level. Amgen, on the other hand, continued such studies. The company's decision to continue this research was consistent with its overall aggressive marketing stance. Pushing the cancer patients' hemoglobin to new heights would have been worth billions in new sales.

The FDA, too, was taking notice, largely because the agency's head of oncology, Richard Pazdur, is a natural skeptic who concluded that the studies pointed to overuse of these drugs, and their potential dangers. Pazdur is a fine scientist and physician, but you don't have to be either to recognize the signs of system failures in medicine.

In the case of hemoglobin-boosting drugs, none of us really knew how to establish uniform hemoglobin targets that would hold for all patients. We didn't know what was normal, what the target should be. We had no idea what dose of these drugs to use and when it made sense to stop pumping it into patients. If doctors had read the label, they would have learned that the FDA approved these drugs for reducing the risk of blood transfusion in patients with solid tumors treated with chemotherapy. That's it. Not a word was said about treating tiredness, not a word about "cancer fatigue." There was no mystery. We knew the gaps in our knowledge were vast, but doctors kept prescribing anyway, and profiting handsomely.

In 2004, the FDA called a meeting of its advisory committee to discuss Henke's head-and-neck study and Leyland-Jones's BEST. The advisory group, called the Oncologic Drugs Advisory Committee, reviewed the data. I was a member of that committee. At the meeting, some of us vented, and our overarching recommendation was to urge the agency to monitor ongoing studies for further evidence of harm.

It's important to remember what the FDA does and what it doesn't do. The agency approves the indications—the use of drugs. It manages the package insert—the label. It can tell you that a drug can be used to treat a specific disease. It can make sure that advertised claims are consistent with the language of the label. It can issue safety warnings, institute restrictions, revoke indications.

However, the agency is not permitted to regulate the practice of medicine. If doctors want to use a drug in a way that goes beyond the indication on the label, they can do so unimpeded. For example, the agency couldn't regulate the use of high-dose chemotherapy and bone marrow transplantation for breast cancer. This procedure made use of approved drugs. That they were used in lethal doses in conjunction with removal and reintroduction of bone marrow fell under the rubric of the practice of medicine. Similarly hemoglobin-building drugs, called erythropoiesis-stimulating agents (ESAs) were approved drugs. They were approved on thin data because we needed an alternative to blood supply, which was at the time threatened by the AIDS epidemic. At the time of approval, no one even suspected how widely these drugs would be used, or that someone would concoct the idea of pushing a cancer patient's hemoglobin into the "normal" range, whatever that means. Doctors were free to use these drugs as they saw fit even as tangible evidence of harm was starting to emerge.

Sure, the J&J direct-to-consumer advertising campaign promised too much. Unfortunately, the armamentarium of penalties that the FDA can impose on companies that make unfounded claims doesn't include the removal of indication. The agency may send warning letters or, at worst, impose fines. In the heyday of ESAs this wasn't about to happen. Warning letters were exceedingly rare, because in the Bush administration former pharmaceutical-company lawyers were running the enforcement arm of the FDA.

AN uninitiated observer might have thought that misgivings about safety and tumor promotion would have depressed the sales of these drugs. Just the opposite: gross sales of Aranesp and Procrit in oncology jumped from $3.783 billion in 2003 to $4.854 billion in 2006. Most of this explosive growth was due to a spectacularly aggressive marketing campaign for Amgen's Aranesp.

In a 2007 presentation for Wall Street analysts, an Amgen executive explained that the company sold two products: "the red juice" to fight anemia, and "the white juice" to fight neutropenia, a deficiency of white blood cells. If you ran an oncology practice at that time, you needed to be able to buy both kinds of juice at the best possible price—and you were therefore completely beholden to Amgen.

This campaign went far beyond direct-to-consumer ads aimed at convincing patients to ask for treatment. Amgen was offering doctors substantial rebates for bulk purchases, thereby inducing doctors to pump ever-larger amounts of Aranesp into each patient.

I obtained a copy of a 2006 supply agreement between Amgen and an oncology practice. This is a proprietary document that doesn't circulate widely, and you can see why. It states that a practice that made a gross purchase of $422,800 worth of Aranesp in a single quarter stood to get back 18 percent of that amount—$76,100—in a rebate. Practices that made larger purchases could get back up to 21 percent on the purchases they had made. Also, Amgen offered discounts on its other drugs, Neulasta and Neupogen, so-called white juice.

These incentives not only induced practices to abandon Procrit in favor of Aranesp, but also made certain that the sales of hemoglobin and neutropenia drugs grew proportionally. Amgen set its sales targets in dollar amounts of gross purchases, which a marketing expert such as Lilla would tell you is an inducement to increase the dose of the drug, giving more of it to each patient. My colleagues in private practice tell me that they would receive calls from Amgen sales reps, informing them when they were underperforming, i.e., running short of earning the discount points.

Since I am an academic oncologist, my salary is not directly determined by the amount of services I sell. I am paid to treat patients, but I am also paid to teach, conduct research, and publish.

Physicians in private practice—who treat more than three-quarters of cancer patients in the United States—are expected to generate certain revenues, and their take-home pay is usually determined by the amount of medical services and drugs they provide.

With these powerful incentives set in motion, many hospitals and oncology practices in the United States instructed nurses to ask leading questions about "fatigue" with the intent of expanding sales to a growing number of patients and upping the dosage to each patient. In August 2007, during a conference call with investors, an Amgen official introduced a chilling term: an *ESA treatment opportunity*.

What is an *ESA treament opportunity*?

A *treatment opportunity* was Amgen's way of saying "a cancer patient." To increase their earnings, drug companies and doctors set out on a search for treatment opportunities, often forgetting about the sacred trust between doctors and patients.

WHILE Lilla was experiencing a burning sensation under her skin, my colleagues were doing quite well, thank you. A friend of mine suggested with bitter irony that oncologists with kids in college should be allowed to target a hemoglobin level of 13.5 g/dl.

Meanwhile, Lilla still had no reasons to ask questions about her treatment. "I just went along with things and did what I had to do," she recalls. "I was feeling good, the treatment was working, and I was managing the chemo just fine."

In 2006, Lilla met several women affiliated with Share, a New York–based suport group for women with breast and ovarian cancer. Some advocacy groups do what doctors and drug companies tell them to do. Share is different. Share members are hard-nosed New Yorkers who seem to have an unlimited number of ways to make it amply clear that they don't tolerate nonsense.

Initially, Lilla's new friends asked her to help with peer counseling on the Share hotline. She took calls from women whose experiences with metastatic breast cancer were similar to her own.

Lilla loved counseling. "You pick up the phone, and somebody is just devastated because they have this horrendous diagnosis," she recalls. "You sit down and talk to them for a few minutes on the phone, and, for one thing, they hear that you are a survivor and that makes them feel good to talk to someone who has made it through. And then they tell you about their emotional or medical concerns. In most cases, if they have medical issues, I suggest a second opinion. When I finished each day, I felt that I had gotten much more than I had given."

Specifically, Lilla got a sense of how the US medical care system operated, not just in New York, but around the country. For some reason, the stories that scared her the most originated in Florida. She realized that these stories fit into broad categories.

There was the story about an uninsured or underinsured woman getting a breast-cancer diagnosis only to realize that she cannot get care. The Centers for Disease Control and Prevention run a free screening program that pays for treating cancers diagnosed through screening. Unfortunately, in most states the program runs out of money on the sixth or seventh month of the fiscal year. CDC says it can pay for care for only 18 percent of eligible patients.

Another category of horror stories stemmed from my colleagues' failure to keep up with the literature. These were shocking accounts of crappy care and deadly ignorance. Failure to prescribe the drug Herceptin to patients who could clearly benefit from it figured prominently on Lilla's list. (Herceptin is used to treat early-stage breast cancers that have receptors for the human epidermal growth factor receptor 2.)

Other callers were women who had exhausted all treatment options. Everything had been tried and nothing worked. Now they wanted to go on a clinical trial, but no trial would have them. They were heavily pretreated, and companies that developed drugs would rather prove efficacy in patients who haven't had a lot of treatment.

In 2003, to make it possible to vacation in Sicily, Lilla had to have two treatments with Herceptin and another drug, Navelbine, while in Italy.

For this, an Italian clinic billed her as a private patient. The Herceptin bill was 640 euros, which at the time translated to $717. In the United States, the hospital billed the insurer between $1,600 and $2,400 for these same drugs.

As an economist, Lilla's husband, Anthony, is interested in innovation and technological change. Before leaving academia—he earned a PhD at the University of Pennsylvania and taught at the University of Connecticut—he was particularly interested in medical technology. Tony is so amazed at the pricing disparity that he uses it as an example in the global-marketing class he teaches at Columbia University. When neither the government nor private payers in the United States care about drug prices, prices careen out of control.

Tony's observation is consistent with the findings of a 2007 report by McKinsey Global Institute. In the United States, the prices of top-selling drugs were 2.3 times higher than in other nations. Overall, costs of branded drugs in the United States are 70 percent higher than in other industrialized countries.

A trip to Canada can save a patient 60 percent on branded drugs.

This is not about the invisible hand of the market. It's the exact opposite.

IN the spring of 2007, Lilla is invited to attend Project LEAD, a four-day residential course taught by the National Breast Cancer Coalition, a Washington umbrella group of which Share is a board member.

LEAD is an acronym for "leadership, education, and advocacy

development." The course teaches skills needed to interpret medical literature, distinguishing solid science from scientific nonsense. The course is about scientific rigor, good public policy, and insistence on good quality of care.

Lilla thinks Project LEAD will make her a better peer counselor. But at the end of the course when she is asked how she would apply her newly earned expertise, Lilla is uncertain. Everything she learns is intellectually enriching and potentially helpful in counseling. If a patient has a question about a particular toxicity or about efficacy of screening for relatives, Lilla will be prepared to answer in depth. Yet, the politics of breast cancer is not among causes to which she is willing to devote the remainder of her life.

In May 2007, Lilla goes to a monthly seminar for graduates of Project LEAD. The seminar is run by two Share activists, Musa Mayer and Helen Schiff. Mayer, daughter of the New York School painter Philip Guston, combines a relaxed attitude with nearly encyclopedic knowledge of breast cancer. Schiff is a classic leftist activist, the sort they don't make anymore. She spent years as a factory worker and union organizer, then, after breast-cancer diagnosis, applied the same urgency to her new political struggle. (Later, Schiff would take a sabbatical from breast-cancer activism to devote more time to advocating for the rights of Israeli Arabs and Palestinians.)

At the seminar, Musa and Helen hand out a stack of back issues of *The Cancer Letter,* a weekly newsletter read by cancer doctors, scientists, and politicized patients. Starting in January 2007, *The Cancer Letter* published a barrage of stories chronicling the emerging evidence on toxicity and tumor promotion associated with ESAs. *The Cancer Letter*'s biggest scoop was learning that a study in Denmark had confirmed the results the German researcher Henke had reported in 2003. Now, the FDA was paying ever-more-careful attention, as were the Centers for Medicare & Medicaid Services, as were congressional investigators. The skeptics were feeling vindicated.

"The FDA will be holding a hearing on these drugs, probably to place them in some kind of a restrictive-access program," Schiff says. "Why don't you testify?"

"Testify? That's the last thing I am prepared to do. I just finished Project LEAD a month ago."

But Schiff regards Lilla's case as a perfect illustration of systemic failure in medicine, and she is not about to let go. The case is all the more astonishing because Lilla is so savvy, so willing to question her doctors. Moreover, Lilla was not facing these decisions alone. She consulted her husband, Tony, every step of the way. (He is so involved and supportive that he later starts a Share group for men whose partners are going through breast and ovarian cancer.)

"Well, why don't you read some of these studies and see if you still feel the same way about testifying?" Schiff suggests.

At home, Lilla reads the stack of papers, old issues of *The Cancer Letter* and a package of studies that appeared in *The New England Journal of Medicine*. The materials all tell the same story: these drugs are leading patients to serious complications, worsening of disease, or death.

Lilla read through the stories systematically, issue after issue. "I was just astounded that I had never heard of any risks or any dangers," she said. "I said, 'Oh my gosh, I had so many of these shots.'"

After reading the papers, Lilla calls Schiff and says, "Yes, I definitely do have to testify."

Chapter 7

Tumor Promotion

I MEET LILLA on May 10, 2007, at a session of the FDA Oncologic Drugs Advisory Committee. She is there to testify at a public-hearing portion of the meeting. I am there as a member of the committee as it gathers to help the agency decide whether new evidence on Aranesp and Procrit justifies instituting restrictions on the way these drugs are used.

Imagine a large table with doctors and scientists arguing about data. If you bother to read up on the science, it can be as passionate as a bar brawl.

It seems half of Wall Street slums at cheap hotels in Rockville, Maryland, where meetings like this are held. This meeting is even farther from D.C. than usual, in a suburb called Germantown. The stock analysts are there in order to feel any turning of the tides and be the first to dump, acquire, or short.

Billions of dollars in trades hinge on the words of the doctors and the scientists with pocket protectors full of sharp pencils. Recommendations from this committee can change a drug's label, influencing doctors' beliefs and altering prescribing patterns and, ultimately, sales.

The presentations that day make me feel particularly good about having protected my patients from unnecessary treatment with red-blood-cell-building drugs. Overtreatment with the drugs under discussion may have been beneficial to doctors, their employers, and the pharmaceutical industry. But now the data are in, one frightening study after another, showing that millions of patients had been exposed to harm.

I was fortunate to have been immune from concerns about billing and revenues. Perhaps I was doubly fortunate because accumulation of wealth is not one of my top 10 goals, and a display of wealth doesn't make it even into the top 250. My car at the time was a rat-gray 1985 Toyota Camry with peeling trim and a fragile air-conditioning system. The thing was an insult to doctors' parking lots, but I felt good about driving it.

THE FDA now stands poised to act. Would the ESA debacle be handled decorously—in a measured scientific debate? Would all the greed and misrepresentations be forgot and this shameful chapter portrayed as an orderly evolution of knowledge, as opposed to what it was—a massive systemic failure?

Red-blood-cell-building agents were anything but an exotic little treatment for a rare disease. These drugs had enormous impact. The committee was about to discuss a group of products that generated the largest revenues in all of oncology. Would the press understand the enormity of what was at stake?

Few reporters understand science. Fewer still have the patience and support of their editors and the space needed to explain complicated issues. The easiest thing to do is to write a story where "experts disagree." This genre of stories persists even in situations where dueling opinions are equally irrelevant. What matters the most are the data, and now the data are in hand. Would an important lesson filter out of this room and into the public consciousness? Would the public and the medical profession hold those at fault accountable? Or would a teaching moment be lost?

AFTER dispassionate analysis is completed and all the facts are laid bare on the table, emotion can rule. Forget subtlety, forget decorum, forget dogma, loyalties, niceties, sacred cows. That's the lesson I learned from the Reverend George R. Follen in September 1973, on my first day at the University of Detroit Jesuit High School.

The Reverend George R., as he liked to be called, taught freshman theology. He sounded like James Cagney even while peppering his speech with biblical Hebrew and ancient Greek. A crew cut added just the right accent for his bulldog face and his mighty rectangular physique.

His first lecture was entirely barked out: "What to expect, gentle-

men . . . Victor Frankl . . . *Man's Search for Meaning* . . ." The course was
a nexus of history, philosophy, and psychology, taught under the broad
rubric of theology.

"From the psychological point of view, gentlemen, the greatest word
in the English language starts with a soft *s*, builds up onto that *h*, then an
i, like the squealing of car brakes. And then if you hit that hard *t*, it's like
slamming your fist into a wall!" For emphasis, the pugilistic priest slammed
his right fist into his left palm, shouting, *"Shit!"*

Then, while continuing to slam his fist into his open hand, the Reverend George R. commenced to jump. "Shit! Shit! Shit! Isn't this wonderful, gentlemen? Shit! Shit! Shit!"

I was thirteen years old, and the Reverend George R. was unlike any
priest I had seen.

At home, my parents asked me how school went, and I said it went
fine. I had to be vague. They would not have understood the enormity of
the lesson the Reverend George R. taught me that day: call things by their
proper name, if only to make yourself feel better.

The Reverend George R. believed that there is right and there is wrong,
and that wisdom can be imparted in the form of maxims. Some of his
teachings were narrow, practical, bordering on the trivial: you cannot
properly read a textbook without marking up the margins. The rest of
his topics were big, very big, intended to guide us though life's perils.
Every time he addressed the class, I felt as if he were addressing me, Otis
Webb Brawley, directly. It seemed that he had somehow gained intimate
knowledge of all the things that terrified me, and the things that stirred
my soul. Sometimes he would take me aside for a private talk, and surely
he realized how grateful I was for this older white man's counsel of a young
black man.

The Reverend George R. told me what to expect. Also, he told me how
to deal with the unknown. What is the proper time to stand tall regardless
of consequences? When do you have the obligation to dodge the bullets?

On the way back to the ghetto, on a Detroit bus, I wrote down the
maxims that would shape my life:

"You have a fire in the belly, do not let it go out. You must constantly
search for fuel for it."

"Be a man for others. Find work where you can make a difference. Use your God-given gifts to improve the lot of others. Always focus on improving the lot of others. Do this for the greater glory of God."

"Be binary, know right and wrong. Be truthful. Have the courage to speak truth to power."

"Never worry about people thinking you are different. Realize, people, both black and white, will try to discourage you. They will try to get at your confidence. They will try to get at your self-confidence."

"You will be tested. Always know your subject matter better than anyone else. You must be good. You must stand up to scrutiny."

"Do not let the naysayers make you feel that you cannot do something. They will call you arrogant. They will call you aloof. They will question your intelligence. They will call you nigger. They will try to assassinate your character. If you are very successful, some will threaten your safety. Spite them by succeeding. It is all right to take satisfaction in your success and their disappointment."

"Do not tolerate fools. Don't compromise on excellence."

"Never let people put you down."

"Feel sorry for people who see no challenges to overcome. Feel sorry for the selfish. Feel sorry for fools. You should feel sorry for a lot of white people. Remember you have character they cannot understand. Relish that you have overcome challenges they could never overcome."

As I prepared for the May 2007 meeting of the FDA Oncologic Drugs Advisory Committee, I hatched a plan that I believed would have impressed the Reverend George R. The day before the FDA meeting, as a courtesy, I informed the Emory public relations department that (1) I intended to set off a pedagogical equivalent of a daisy cutter, and (2) I didn't give a shit what they thought and would do what I thought was right regardless of consequences.

Before the FDA advisory committee begins deliberations, members of the public are allowed to testify. The American Society of Clinical Oncology and a Texas-based company called US Oncology are lobbying against additional restrictions on ESAs. The patients who come to testify that day feel otherwise.

It's a pleasure to see Carolina Hinestrosa, a beautiful forty-nine-year-old Latina who had survived two bouts of breast cancer. Carolina, vice president of the National Breast Cancer Coalition, delivers polished speeches that I agree with in at least nine cases out of ten. And on the tenth case, our disagreements are respectful.

"We believe that as a community—scientists, clinicians, regulators, manufacturers, patients, and society—we need to learn what really works for women with and at risk for breast cancer to make sure that knowledge is incorporated into clinical practice," Carolina says that day. "We must also figure out what it costs us, healthwise and financially, to make fully informed determinations of what is acceptable and appropriate care. There is an underlying trust patients and consumers have in scientists, doctors, and the FDA regulators to look after their best interests as you evaluate the benefits and harms of the drugs, tests, and all interventions that become available to fight cancer.

"Consumers trust the system to offer interventions that are based on high-quality evidence, and appropriately designed randomized trials are the gold standard to obtain evidence of benefits and harms for all interventions, therapeutic or supportive."

Yes, yes, yes, and yes, I scribble in my briefing book. Carolina understands epidemiology, she understands public health, she understands biostatistics. Her advocacy is genuine. There is no posturing, no angling for political advantage or an "unrestricted" grant that drug companies hand out to friendly patient-advocate groups.

Later I would learn that Carolina was battling a sarcoma, a cancer of connective tissue, caused by radiation treatment she received as part of breast-cancer therapy. She would succumb to that disease at age fifty.

Lilla is next at the microphone:

"Over the course of years of treatment—with only one short 'chemo vacation'—I have had many doses of Procrit and then Aranesp. The recent discussion of the risks in using these anemia drugs has caused me considerable worry. In the case of these drugs, we believe that they stimulate oxygenation, but in stimulating the blood cells have we also stimulated and encouraged the cancer cells? Have the growth factors that were assumed to help avoid blood transfusions and the effects of anemia led to

tumor progression instead? Does the increased risk of blood clots outweigh the alleged benefits of having greater levels of energy? How is it
possible that what was meant to help me might have actually made things
worse?"

These are excellent points, which I agree with wholeheartedly, but I
also see that they need amplification. The advocates in the room are being technical and not speaking in sound bites. It's up to me—a techno-
crat with a pocket protector—to let loose a real zinger that will make
the press and the public understand that this is not an obscure scientific
controversy. I have the standing—the gravitas—to commence jumping
and shouting, "Shit! Shit! Shit!"

As the committee moves to discussion of the data, I summarize the
emerging studies that suggest that these drugs stimulate cancer growth.
"I'm concerned that this compound is a stimulant, a 'tumor fertilizer,'
for epidermal tumors," I say. "What data do you have to assure me that
this is not Miracle-Gro for cancer?"

Of course, I realize that the question is a variation on "When did you
stop beating your wife?" But why shouldn't punishment for profiting
from tumor growth include a challenge to prove the negative?

Any reporter who ignores this question would probably also be able
to block out a jumping, fist-slamming, "Shit!"-screaming Jesuit. My question ends up on the front page of *The New York Times* as well as in almost
every news story covering the meeting.

IN 2010—two years after the committee meeting—the FDA placed new,
tough restrictions on these drugs. The restrictions say that ESAs are not to
be given in settings where the goal is to cure the patient. Breast and head-
and-neck cancers are now listed as diseases where these drugs are best
avoided. Every time doctors administer these drugs, they are required to
explain the risks to patients and document that a discussion of risks has
taken place.

Lilla's disease is kept under control for a decade after it turned metastatic. Every time her hemoglobin drops too low, she opts for a blood
transfusion rather than an ESA. (Transfusions should be given in place
of ESAs whenever feasible, particularly to patients with metastatic dis-

ease. A patient with active disease is more likely to suffer tumor progression: the more tumor you have, the more tumor there is to stimulate.) Lilla learns that she can live comfortably when her hemoglobin drops.

"I have mentioned to my doctor that at 10 g/dl, I do very well. At nine, I do well. At eight, I do well. It's when it gets below eight is when I need a transfusion," she said. "I would have been absolutely fine. I would not have needed anything."

In my opinion doctors who prescribed ESAs to patients like Lilla Romeo were not treating actual patients. They were treating numbers on charts, and such treatment was both costly and harmful.

The exact magnitude of harm is harder to gauge. In the aggregate, about $37 billion went to pay for these drugs in oncology between 1996 and 2009. It's now safe to say that most of that money was spent on drugs that were prescribed for the wrong reasons and under false, manufactured pretenses. These drugs were not used to cure disease or make patients feel better. They were used to make money for doctors and pharmaceutical companies at the expense of patients, insurance companies, and taxpayers.

The technical term for this is overtreatment, and overtreatment equals harm. I can't stop wondering how many mammograms these resources could have bought for people like Edna Riggs.

As we were gathering information for this book, Lilla requested copies of her medical records from the doctors who had treated her and learned that she had received a lot more Procrit and Aranesp than she knew.

"I hope you are sitting down," she said in an e-mail sent before she entered a home hospice. "I asked for the original flow sheets and got the shock of my life. My first dose was administered 1/11/01 and almost weekly thereafter. All and all, I was given 221 1/2 doses."

"Flow sheets" are the spreadsheets that oncologists use to keep track of the dose and date of administered anticancer drugs. They showed that Lilla received nearly six times the number of doses she thought she received. Was this medical malpractice? Not at all. The oncologists who gave Lilla these drugs were practicing medicine in accordance with widely accepted standards. The problem was, those standards sucked.

Hemoglobin-building drugs contributed $400,000 to $600,000 to

Lilla's bill alone. Certainly, if these drugs weren't available, Lilla would have needed some transfusions, but she would not have needed them until her hemoglobin dropped below 8 g/dl, rather than the arbitrary level decreed by doctors.

The cost of these drugs may have been more profound than money. They may have shortened Lilla's life. This shouldn't surprise anyone. When the entire medical—and political—system turns a blind eye to evidence and errs on the side of financial self-interest, people like Lilla pay.

Chapter 8

Defibrillation

AS A MEDICAL STUDENT at the University of Chicago in the 1980s, I craved the experience of ER duty. The ER seemed to be the kind of place to flourish as a badass for the forces of good: racing against the clock to stop gushing bleeds, administering shocks to get hearts to beat again, palpating the divide separating life from death.

In the beginning of my residency at the University Hospitals Case Medical Center in Cleveland, I loved the ER—the quick interactions with patients, working six cases at a time, running from room to room. I got to stitch. I got to put in central lines and stick needles into body cavities to draw out fluid.

The ER is also the slimy underbelly of the system, the place where its flaws are at their most visible.

SAUL Greenberg's chart identifies him as a fifty-seven-year-old white male, but that tells only a small part of the story. Saul is the sort of older Jewish guy you might see wearing white patent-leather loafers with a matching belt, an ensemble known as the Full Cleveland, which is, of course, perfectly appropriate for a guy living in Cleveland.

The Full Cleveland is conjecture on my part. When I see Saul, he is in a hospital gown. He is also wearing a massive gold chain and a large, dark brown toupee. When you work ER, you look at fingernails a lot, they can tell you a lot about a patient. Saul's are meticulously manicured, finished in clear lacquer that throws off considerable sheen.

Saul cultivates the appearance of a dangerous man, a Meyer Lansky. He drinks a lot, smokes, hires hookers. His chart says he has bipolar disorder. Saul has also been declared disabled by the federal government and is one of the few people I have ever met who receives Medicare before reaching sixty-five.

Saul's second major medical problem is heart disease. He has had several heart attacks, and his heart has rhythm problems. He will regularly go into ventricular tachycardia, rapid heart rhythm stemming from the ventricles of the heart. His blood pressure will drop, and he will pass out. This event is often called sudden death, or SD. If Saul is not shocked out of it quickly or if he doesn't get CPR until he gets shocked out of it, he is certain to die.

Since Saul has Medicare, he is able to get an expensive medical device, one of the first mass-produced implantable defibrillators. Saul has this contraption placed in his abdomen, with wires running up to his heart. On a chest X-ray, you can see the small paddles near his heart. If his heart goes into tachycardia, his defibrillator will fire, shocking him out of it.

Today, defibrillators are small—roughly the size of a railroad watch. They go in the chest, and implanting them takes relatively minor surgery. In 1987, defibrillators were much larger, and implantation required a significant operation.

Saul comes to my ER because his defibrillator has fired. He is moved to the head of the triage line and is put on a monitor in a cardiac resuscitation room. I get called away from other patients to see him. The defibrillator is a new entity and we already know that we will have to call the cardiologist on call as soon as I finish my initial evaluation.

I give Saul my standard greeting: "I am Otis Brawley. I am one of the doctors here. How can I help you?" (This introduction, which reflects my aversion to titles, is a career-long quirk. Being a doctor is my function in life. Yet, I cringe at the *Dr.* before my name. Friends who noticed this have nicknamed me Dr. Call-Me-Otis.)

In a jovial tone, Saul tells me that he has a defibrillator and that it has gone off.

"When?"

"Two hours ago."

"What were you doing?"

"Well, Doc, I was with this pro, and I came to the magic moment, and I was tensing up, and I must have had a rhythm problem. I must have gone out, 'cause all I remember is waking up hearing her say, 'Wow! Are you for real!' It was great, Doc, and I didn't even have to pay her. She didn't charge me because I charged her, so to speak."

It takes me a minute to realize—or, perhaps, accept—that Saul is telling me that the prostitute felt the shock of his defibrillator going off. Did she feel the shock because of the proximity of their bodies? Did penetration play a role?

I kind of want to know and I kind of don't.

CEDRIC Jones is a twenty-three-year-old black man. He is well built, muscular. He looks like a college athlete, but isn't. Cedric is a frequent flier at the University Hospitals ER. He was born with a malformed heart. Doctors corrected the condition, called tetralogy of Fallot, with a series of surgeries during his childhood. He can function normally, except occasionally his heart develops a rhythm problem.

Cedric will go into ventricular tachycardia, a racing heart rate that begins in the heart's lower chamber. But unlike most people who have this condition, his body maintains a good blood pressure, and he doesn't pass out. When he feels that his heart isn't beating right, he knows that it is time to get to the hospital.

Cedric has no insurance and has to use the ER for all his health care. Will any insurer write a policy for a guy with Cedric's chronic problems? No way, not in 1987. He is in a particularly bizarre conundrum: he has no job and lives with his parents. This makes him too wealthy for Medicaid. His parents have insurance, but it stopped covering him after he turned eighteen. Cedric tells me that he has lost every job he ever had because he is constantly in and out of the hospital.

Cedric comes to the ER once every two months, give or take. In an ER, where foul language is as commonplace as knife wounds, Cedric stands out. He is a nice young man, drug-free, clean-cut, pleasant, polite. The permanent nurses greet him and he knows them by name. Even doctors on ER rotation get to meet him at least once.

I meet Cedric during one of his visits. He has told the triage nurse
that he is in ventricular tachycardia and needs cardioversion—electric
shock. He knows what he needs better than anyone else.

This nurse is relatively new to the ER. She doesn't believe him. It
makes no sense for a clean-cut, muscular, young black man to come in
and ask for cardioversion. A junkie might develop all sorts of cardiac
problems at an early age, but Cedric is clearly not a junkie. What is this
young man doing asking for cardioversion? The idea that he can be in
V-tach and be walking and talking is even more unbelievable. And why
does he be talk about it with the easy confidence of a physician?

Yet, because Cedric is so well-spoken, the nurse finally takes him seriously and puts him on a monitor in the cardiac room. Later, she tells me
that she nearly fainted when she saw the rhythm: classic ventricular tachycardia.

The nurse calls me immediately. My attending, who is down the hall,
knows Cedric. She is busy and tells me to handle it: "He needs cardioversion. He'll tell you how he wants it done."

I examine Cedric quickly, as a nurse inserts an IV in his arm.

"I am still a little afraid of the pain of being shocked," Cedric says
apologetically.

I promise that I will put him under.

"Could you give me two hundred joules of electricity? That's what I
usually need." Also, Cedric says that he wants 15 mg of Versed, a
Valium-like drug with a short half-life.

Now, 15 mg is a whole lot of Versed. "That's at least five times the dose
I am used to giving," I object. I explain that this much drug could cause
respiratory depression, which is doctor-speak for cessation of breathing.

He nods. He knows.

"If that happens, we would have to breathe for you with the Ambu
bag for a while," I keep objecting. An Ambu bag is a self-inflating bag
used in resuscitation.

Cedric assures me that we will not have to. He knows the dose that
works. He begs me to make sure that he is out when I shock him because two hundred joules will hurt so bad. He is literally crying, plead-

ing to be out. He has been hurt before. I promise him that I will make sure he is out.

I don't get around to telling him that two hundred is a lot of joules. Usually, you start with one hundred, or even fifty. You go up only if that doesn't work. But the attending was clear: "Cedric will tell you what to do."

Three nurses are in the room. One of them starts pushing the Versed into IV tubing, which has half-normal saline running at 120 cc per minute. Another starts shaving hair off his chest for the paddles. I continue talking back and forth with Cedric as he begs me to make sure he will be out.

I hear him, but I stop the nurse at 10 mg and assess the situation. Cedric is still talking. I give the nurse the go-ahead to give more as I worry about the dose. Cedric stops talking and seems to fall asleep.

I feel his pulse. It is still strong. I can see his heartbeat. It is V-taching at a rate of 140 per minute. One nurse has an Ambu bag as we all watch his chest move. We count every breath.

I charge the machine to two hundred joules, per Cedric's instructions.

I place one paddle on the anterior chest and the other on the side of the left chest under the armpit.

I call out, *"Clear!"* I look to make sure the nurses aren't touching the steel hospital bed. I press the trigger, firing two hundred joules into Cedric's body.

As his body absorbs the massive shock, Cedric emits a scream, a loud, long, shrieking scream: *"Nigger!!!!!"*

Startled, I look at Cedric, then at the nurses. I feel uneasy, but I am clearly less distressed than these three white women. The intensity of Cedric's scream has startled me, not the word he screamed. (Sure, it's wrong for a white to call a black by that name, but Cedric is black. So, it's okay, almost. In my childhood neighborhood, we called each other nigger as a form of endearment. I haven't encountered an occasion to let this word roll off my tongue over a couple of decades, which doesn't necessarily mean that I never will.)

I am sure Cedric didn't intend the word as a term of endearment. Horrific pain was his evidence that I disregarded his specific instructions and skimped on the elephant dose of Versed he needed.

I compose myself enough to make certain that the procedure was successful. Cedric is in normal sinus rhythm. I watch his respiration.

After about ten minutes, Cedric wakes up. Will he remember the pain or the scream? One beautiful thing about massive doses of benzodiazepines is their ability to cause amnesia.

"How are you feeling?" I ask calmly.

Mercifully, Cedric doesn't remember the pain of the electric shock. He tells me that I am cool. "Never had a black doctor do a cardioversion." He is back to his old well-spoken, pleasant self.

We admit him overnight and discharge him from a monitored bed the next day. He comes by the ER on the way home to say thanks to the nurses and me, as he does after every visit.

Cedric needs the same implantable defibrillator that Saul has. Saul qualifies for Medicare, which paid for the device. Cedric has no insurance and no hope. Indeed, if Cedric tries to get private insurance, he will be rejected as uninsurable due to a preexisting condition. He gets his care from the ER, and the hospital never collects any money for the care it provides. All the insured patients who come to the hospital subsidize his care, which would be less expensive if he had a regular doctor and gets the defibrillator he needs.

I hear about Cedric's subsequent trips to the ER for the remaining two years I am in Cleveland, but I never learn what happened to him after I left. I hope he got one of those newer, low-voltage implantable defibrillators, but I know that it's more likely that he died hoping for one.

Untimely death isn't even the most horrifying aspect of the story of Saul and Cedric. Scarier still is that in this story, medical technology is the only thing that has changed. The disparities between the insured and the uninsured remain. Likely, they increase as technology improves.

Chapter 9

Palpitation

I ENCOUNTER NORMA SHEVCHENKO at an ER examination room at the University Hospitals Case Medical Center in October 1986. The triage nurse places Norma in the cardiac section, and my job is to determine whether she is having a heart attack.

According to the forms Norma Shevchenko fills out to be admitted, she is fifty-six. She has not changed into an examination gown either because the nurse had forgotten to tell her to or because she missed or disregarded the instructions. This is an inconvenience—much of the physical exam will have to wait—but seeing her in street clothes gives me some clues about what ails Norma. I see that the hour notwithstanding—it's after 2:00 a.m.—Norma has taken a special effort to pull herself together.

She is wearing a blue dress with a white lace collar, the sort you might see on an older woman at a church service. I note a large cameo brooch; it's ivory, old-world. She has applied eye shadow and a generous daub of perfume. Her thinning hair is dyed uniform raven-black, with no variation from root to tip. As a second-year resident, I know that such observations are important.

Norma is sitting on the examining bench, knees over the edge, forearms on top of the legs. The shoulders are slouchy. The palms are up, with one palm cradled in the other. This, too, is important.

"How are you, Mrs. Shevchenko?" I say.

The name is the most important part of the question. An ER is a chaotic place. Papers get dropped on the floor, things get mixed up, clipboards get placed on the wrong racks. You can't take it for granted that you are talking with the right patient. If the woman in front of me is someone other than Mrs. Shevchenko, this is her opportunity to let me know.

I take the absence of an objection as a sign that I have the right patient. So far, so good.

"I am Otis Brawley, I am one of the doctors here." I extend my hand.

Her handshake is weak. I pause, leaving space for Norma to talk. She doesn't, so I prompt her: "How can I help you?"

"I can feel my heart beating," she says slowly. That's what I see in her chief complaint, but I want to hear it from her directly.

"How bad?"

"Bad."

"Do you have any shortness of breath?"

"Maybe a little."

"Do you have any chest pains?"

She nods. "Some."

Irritation sets in. I am impatient at her slow answers. This can't be helped because Norma and I are machines that run at different speeds. Otis Brawley has to knock out three to four cases an hour, and Norma Shevchenko has all the time in the world.

"Have you had any ankle swelling?"

"Not like last time I came here," she says.

"You've been here before? When?"

"In May, I think."

I note that she was here six months ago—a frequent flier. "What did we tell you then?"

"A young woman doctor told me to use less salt."

"Do you have family history of heart disease?"

"Yes, my husband. Never found out whether it was a stroke or a heart attack."

When we ask about family history, we mean the patient's blood relatives. The goal is to pin down hereditary risk factors, and a husband's history doesn't help. In this case, I realize that I learn something more useful, something about environmental exposures. Her husband's diet—

also, presumably, her diet—could have contributed to his death. This is all I need for now; time is short.

I have Norma roll up a sleeve and check her blood pressure. It's slightly elevated, 157 over 92. You would expect that in someone mildly obese, someone like Norma. I look at the forms and see that she is not diabetic. Not yet.

"How long has it been going on?"

"What?"

"Your feeling the heartbeat."

"I don't know."

"Have you ever experienced this palpitation before?"

"What?"

"The flutter you describe. Have you had it before?"

"I think so. Two weeks ago I just couldn't get out of bed all day."

"Is there anything you can do to make it worse?"

"Why?"

"Does it get worse when you walk faster?"

"No."

"Can you walk across the floor?"

Norma gets off the bench tentatively and looks back at me for approval.

"Are you able to walk up steps?"

She nods.

"How many flights of steps can you walk up?"

"Three," she says after a pause. "Then my hip starts hurting. My right hip."

"What drugs are you taking?"

"Nothing, except for when my hip hurts."

"Have you had any surgery?"

"I had a women's procedure."

"A hysterectomy?"

She nods.

"When?"

"About ten years ago."

I ask Norma whether she has been drinking caffeinated drinks: coffee,

tea, Coke, Pepsi. She hasn't. I ask about less obviously caffeinated drinks:
cream soda, Mountain Dew.

"Do you smoke?"

"Never have."

"Did Mr. Shevchenko?"

"Three packs a day."

I am fishing. I have no idea what to do with this information. Of
course, I suspect that living for decades with a three-pack-a-day smoker
can't be good for your heart and lungs, but I don't know this. In 1986, no
one does; the studies confirming health hazards for passive smokers
would come years later.

"Do you have children, grandchildren?"

"No."

"Do you go to work?"

She shakes her head from side to side. No.

"Do you belong to a church, a Ukrainian church, maybe?" Ordinarily,
this would be none of my business, but Shevchenko is an obviously Ukrainian name, and the Ukrainian community in Cleveland likely provides
social support for its members.

"No, I am not Ukrainian. John was."

"Well, Mrs. Shevchenko," I say, getting out of the chair, "I'll be back in
a few minutes. Meanwhile, a nurse will have you change and take your
EKG. Then we'll know more about what's wrong with you."

AS a first year-resident at Case Western Reserve University (CWRU) in
1985, I got to pull ER rotations in a sustained manner: twelve hours a day,
six days a week. On those rotations, I encountered a legion of patients like
Norma Shevchenko. Everything I see in Norma tells me what's wrong
with her physically: absolutely nothing.

It's possible that she experienced heart palpitation, but that she dressed
up for a visit to the ER—the lace collar, the cameo brooch—tells me
that in the middle of the night Norma was overcome with excruciating
loneliness and desire to be seen, touched, cared for. Thirsting for social
interaction, she went to the nearest emergency room and ended up in
my care.

In doctor-speak, patients like Norma are known under the nickname *gomer,* short for "get out of my emergency room." The term became ubiquitous after 1978, when it appeared in a novel called *The House of God,* an account of an internship at Beth Israel Medical Center. The novel, by Harvard professor Steve Bergman, writing under the pseudonym Samuel Shem, is about a young man's headfirst dive into the absurdity of real-world medicine. The novel burrows so deep into your consciousness that it starts to fuse with reality, infecting it with crazed lingo. I don't know whether this was the case of life imitating art, but almost all male doctors of my generation claim that their internship was exactly like *The House of God.* Mine was *almost* exactly like that—minus the promiscuous nurses.

In *The House of God,* a gomer is someone who "has lost—often through age—what goes into being a human being."

In the novel, the gomers were demented residents of nursing homes whose bodies wouldn't die. My experience at Case Western showed me other categories of gomers as well. These people were not demented—just starved for companionship and the human touch. About three-quarters of these were female. Women who came to the ER for these reasons were rarely thin. They were almost always widowed. They presented with depressed affect, and they dressed up to see the doctor, even in the middle of the night. The few of them who were thin seemed hyperactive, and when they showed up in the ER, I made a point of sending out their blood to check for thyroid function.

Another category of gomers were little old ladies in their seventies whose chief complaint was constipation. Their physical exam was totally normal, which left you wondering whether they had your garden-variety constipation that a quart of prune juice could clear up, or whether you were dealing with an obstruction from previously undiagnosed colon cancer or a buildup of scar tissue from a C-section performed forty-five years ago.

During my first ER rotation, I realized that on a busy night I would see as many as forty patients, and at least a dozen of them were not physically ill. Once you've recognized that nothing is physically wrong with your patient, your life doesn't get easier. Quite the opposite, it gets harder because (a) you don't know whether you are right or are just missing something, and (b) she just might return to your ER in cardiac arrest forty-five minutes after you told her to go home and rest. Eventually, gomers have to die, and many will experience genuine medical emergencies. You want to make sure that you are not the idiot who sends a dying woman into the night.

To be defensive, it's possible to admit Norma Shevchenko to the hospital, but admitting bullshit patients will quickly make you a pariah among your colleagues. An ER doc who sends every Norma Shevchenko to the ward (or, worse, to cardiac intensive care) becomes known as a Sieve (another *House of God* term). A Sieve has no ability to filter impurities, everything runs through it.

The opposite of a Sieve is a Wall. No gomer gets through a Wall, but you don't want to be a Wall, either, because eventually you'll make a mistake, and a Norma Shevchenko will pay the ultimate price for your determination.

My decisions could have enormous implications on Norma's life. Depending on what I conclude—or what I guess—Norma would end up either in the cardiac intensive care unit or back at the parking lot. Was this what she bargained for when she dressed up to see a doctor in the middle of a particularly distressing night?

As I examine Norma, I perform every test and scientific evaluation I can think of to rule out a cardiac event. Then I perform them all again. The result is unchanged: nothing suspicious.

On the way to see an attending, I keep asking myself whether I missed anything. I can't think of anything. Nothing is obviously physically wrong with this patient. Under *The House of God* nomenclature, Norma is a classic LOL in NAD—a Little Old Lady in No Apparent Distress. She could probably use some psychiatric help, or perhaps simple human companionship will do. I do feel compassion for her, but in my role as a second-year resident on emergency rotation, I can do nothing to ease her despair.

The attending agrees with me. "Another gomer?" she asks after I present the case.

I nod.

"It never ceases to amaze me how these people are just not sick." She signs off on my decision and I return to Norma's examination room. She is still in her examination gown, still hooked up to the EKG monitor, which is still showing a healthy heartbeat.

"Mrs. Shevchenko," I say, and wait for her to look up. "We have checked everything we can think of, and we can't find anything that would make us suspect heart disease."

I am careful to say "we can't find" any heart disease, because that's really all we know. I don't say "you don't have heart disease," because there could be disease we haven't detected, or disease preparing to strike suddenly, without warning.

I've had many patients argue with me when I give them news that would generally be classified as good: there is no reason to think that you have a lethal illness. Luckily, Mrs. Shevchenko doesn't argue. She seems accepting of my diagnosis. It's possible that she got what she wanted: a focused physical examination and confirmation that she is still among the living.

I catch sight of Mrs. Shevchenko leaving the ER. "Oh, shit," I say to the nurse. "What if she returns in cardiac arrest?"

A patient such as Edna Riggs seeking to reattach a breast is very different from a patient such as Norma Shevchenko, whose problems are primarily existential. But they do have one thing in common: their appearance in the ER is an indication of failure of the system. Emergency rooms are the only places in America's health-care system that are legally obliged to care for everyone—and then they get bashed for doing it.

The problem is vast, its cost enormous. Yet, it's studied mostly in snapshots. One of the most intriguing of these snapshots emerged in a study by a group of researchers at New York University and Bellevue Hospital Center. The researchers, led by Maria C. Raven, of NYU, attempted to identify patients like Norma Shevchenko, repeat customers. They identified 139 patients at high risk of returning to emergency rooms at urban public hospitals like Grady between 2001 and 2006.

Mean Medicaid expenditures for these patients were $39,188 and

$84,040 per patient for the years immediately prior to study participation and immediately following it. Perhaps not surprisingly, 56 percent of these patients said that the ER was their usual source of care.

Misuse of the ER is almost never the patient's fault. If you are poor and living in Atlanta's inner city, good luck finding a private primary-care physician. No mammogram for Edna Riggs. As for mental health services—forget it. It's off the table. No psychiatric social worker for Norma Shevchenko.

I admire doctors who are able to thrive in emergency medicine. They put up with excruciating boredom that eats up most of their time for the sake of the adrenaline rush that comes with handling genuine life-and-death cases. They get to save lives, and they are among the finest raconteurs in all of medicine.

Yet, after ER rotations at Case Western, I realized that I couldn't be one of them.

Chapter 10

Saving Mr. Huzjak

FRED HUZJAK'S HANDS tell a story. They are the calloused hands of a steelworker. The rest of seventy-eight-year-old Fred Huzjak is in no condition to engage in storytelling. I would never learn whether he even knew we had met. It's October 1986, and I am a second-year resident in medicine assigned to Hanna House 4 at the University Hospitals of Cleveland.

Mr. Huzjak lies in front of me, obtunded, mentally dulled, eyes open, not responsive to questions. I am not sure how conscious he is. The guys at the ER who first evaluated him determined that he reacts to pain, but that's about it.

Mr. Huzjak was brought to the ER for "failure to thrive," which is another way of saying that he doesn't seem to have any idea of what's going on around him. His daughter brings him in because the family had realized that he had slowly grown unresponsive. This is not unusual. A sick person often does not talk or socialize much, and sometimes it takes the family a little while to realize that the familiar quietness has changed to unresponsiveness.

I look at the charts and see that Mr. Huzjak has a plethora of underlying problems, including a five-month history of Stage IV non-small-cell lung cancer (NSCLC). He was a pack-a-day smoker for forty years and has been treated for chronic obstructive pulmonary disease for the past six years.

The cancer had spread to both lungs, and to his spine, pelvis, and liver. He was treated with cisplatin and VP-16 for four cycles over twelve weeks. (In 1986, that was the standard of care, the best we could do.) The disease progressed while on therapy and treatment was stopped. From that point on, the goal was to manage the symptoms.

Huzjak's dry skin indicates that he is dehydrated. That's because he is too out of it to know that he needs to drink. We can't tell how much of his brain function is still intact. We don't know whether he is able to see or smell or taste or hear. When we ask him to follow a finger with his eyes, he doesn't. He remains inert when we ask, "Mr. Huzjak, can you hear me?" His face is completely placid. Is this because he has no control over facial muscles? Maybe.

His extraocular muscles appear intact, though. His pupils are equal and reactive to light and accommodation. His neck is supple. His lungs have some wheezing-breath sounds. He has bilateral pleural effusions, fluid in the chest cavity. This is common in lung cancer and prevents the lung from fully expanding. He seems to respond only to noxious stimuli (medicalese for pain we cause in examination). Labs show that his white blood count is 10.3 with a slight left shift. This is doctor-speak for evidence of infection.

The systems in Huzjak's body are failing in a relentless, rapid cascade.

IN a big university hospital, you have patients who have private attending physicians and patients "on the service." Patients who are on the service don't have a regular doctor. They are almost always admitted through the ER and usually are poor and under- or uninsured. They get care from the residents, with some input from an attending designated by the medicine department for the month. At CWRU, we take pride in giving these folks extraordinary care. Huzjak has a private physician, Jim Claren, a good guy, whom we residents like.

We enter Huzjak's room and introduce ourselves to the patient even though we know he can't respond. You always work to show respect to the patient. In the case of Huzjak, introducing ourselves may not help the patient, but it helps the family, or so you hope. We introduce ourselves to the patient's daughter, too.

I go through my usual introduction.

That day I have a team of two interns, Beth and Tony.

We ask Huzjak's daughter what occurred over the past week. She confirms the history: lung cancer that grew through chemotherapy, then, recently, social withdrawal.

We examine Huzjak and verify what we have been told by our colleagues in the ER and by his daughter. When we finish gathering all the data, it's 5:30 a.m. I suggest to the interns that we wait till 6:00 a.m. to call Claren, Huzjak's private physician. Even though we didn't get any sleep, it's better not to wake an attending for a nonemergency, especially if he is a decent attending who doesn't abuse us. At 6:15, we page Claren and he calls back almost immediately.

Beth presents the patient as I listen in on a second phone. Claren remembers the history, a sign of a good doc.

"What do you suggest?" Claren says.

Beth notes that we had started Huzjak on three antibiotics. The goal is to drain the effusion. We are hydrating him by IV and watching for fluid overload. Claren agrees.

We can't do a thing about the root cause of Mr. Huzjak's problems: the galloping lung cancer. This man is near death, and we have to accept that we are helpless to stop it. Allowing him to exit with dignity would be the only responsible, the only humane, thing to do.

Claren says he had repeatedly tried to get a DNR—a "do not resuscitate" order—from the daughter. He tried at every office visit and every hospital admission after it became clear that the drugs weren't doing any good. Efforts along these lines are called "hanging out black crepe"— they are to lower expectations, prepare the family for bad news. Alas, Huzjak's daughter is determined to hang on to hope.

In part, this is about our culture. As Americans, we are a never-give-up, pull-yourself-up-by-your-bootstraps kind of people. To us, death is a failure of medicine. Death has to be somebody's fault, and we are generous in assigning the blame. This ideology is unfair to patients who, as we say, "fail" therapies. And it's unfair to doctors, who fall short of producing miraculous cures. Unable to accept the inevitability of death, we can't make plans, can't talk reasonably about our preferences for the circumstances of our passing and about what we want to happen after we are gone.

I wonder whether the Huzjak family's denial of reality is in part caused by their reaction to Claren. He is patrician, a person from a planet different from theirs. His country-club sport coats, his bow ties, his penny loafers with dimes in place of pennies, are images the Huzjaks may find intimidating. He is a good, compassionate doc, but maybe his message is coming through as patronizing, or simply hard to relate to.

Might class be larger than race for the Huzjaks? Would the difficult message be heard if it came from a young black man who came up the hard way, who faced the same hardships they face every day? It's worth a try.

"Would you allow me to talk with her?" I ask Claren. (You don't meddle with a private's patient without his permission.)

"Be my guest," he says. "Just remember, the daughter has unreasonable expectations." He tells us that she was upset when Claren declined to give further chemotherapy, and she said no to hospice care.

Claren's situation would have been easier had she simply fired him. He would have been off the hook. Yet she did nothing of the sort. She let the doctor stay on the case, but rejected his recommendations. She did not even get a second opinion.

When I arrive at Huzjak's room, his daughter is in a chair, asleep. I gently awaken her. She is in her forties, obviously tired, obviously distressed. I tell her that I know that this is a difficult time for her. I tell her Mr. Huzjak reminds me a lot of my father. I tell her that I have had to deal with my father's illness, which was similar to Huzjak's. My father, too, was a World War II vet, and he, too, had NSCLC and had a rough course with it.

I tell her that Huzjak is stable for now, but his condition will change over the next few days, and some decisions should be made.

"I would like you to talk with my brothers," she says.

There is hope.

We agree to meet at 8:30 a.m., and I arrange for her to have a phone and some privacy.

AT 8:30 a.m. I enter Huzjak's room and meet his two sons. They are in their forties. Also, I meet the wife of a son and the husband of the daughter, and one grandson. Something tells me that the sons, like their father, work in the steel mills. I had recently watched the movie *Deer Hunter,* which was set in part among Slavic steelworkers from a rust-belt town. I asked one of the nurses. Huzjak is a Croatian name.

I explain that we are working with Claren, that he will be in later in the day, and that he asked me to talk with the family. I explain the extent of Huzjak's lung cancer. It's in the liver, both lungs, the mediastinum (the chest between the lungs), pelvis, ribs, and spinal bones. We are concerned that it has spread to his brain (we'd need to do studies to find out for sure). He has already received the best chemotherapy we have, and the disease grew despite it. The cancer is progressing, and nothing can be done to halt it.

The disease has caused complications, which include pleural effusion, fluid in the chest, which keeps the lungs from expanding. We are concerned about pericardial effusion, fluid around the heart, which can negatively affect the pumping action of the heart muscle. His lungs are not functioning well. He may have pneumonia, which may be due to an obstruction in his bronchial tree, the windpipes. I explain that when cancer narrows the windpipes, we often see an infection. Pneumonia is frequently the immediate cause of death.

"We need to decide what is reasonable," I say. "We need in whatever we do to stress comfort for Mr. Huzjak."

I speak slowly, deliberately. I know that every poorly chosen word can and will work against me. After long hours of running from one task to another, I have to change speeds, I have to slow down, I have to demonstrate compassion, express it as clearly as I can. I have to understand where they are coming from and get to the fundamental cause of their resistance to accepting death as a final destination for a sick man. Death in this case is not a failure of the system.

I know how much is riding on this conversation. If it goes well, this family will bid farewell to Huzjak. If it goes badly, this man will suffer through a plethora of procedures that can only do harm.

I lay out the multiple-choice problem before us. We must pick one of three possible options.

I start with the most absurd: We perform diagnostic studies and treat all of these problems. This will cause their father and grandfather a lot of discomfort at best, agony at worst. We will not be able to control the pain with anaesthesia. I explain that Huzjak's respiratory system is fragile. Drugs that control pain also decrease the respiratory drive in his brain. Narcotics that control the pain also bring closer the day when he will be put on a ventilator, and once he is on it, there he will stay until his last breath.

I go through the list of invasive procedures that are in store for Huzjak: a scope placed through his mouth and on into his lungs to look for pneumonia and obstruction, tubes placed into his chest, spinal taps, and possibly even medicines injected into his chest and spine. These *may* prolong his life—briefly.

May is the key word. Since we can't assess him neurologically, I can't say how far gone he is. I don't even know whether he is conscious. Has his cerebrum stopped functioning? Is he driven only by his brain stem? I know that he screams from pain, but I have no idea whether this is a primal response or evidence of more complex brain processing.

Without question, we will increase his suffering, but the result will not change. He will have widely metastatic, untreatable cancer from which he will die.

The second approach—which the medical team and Claren favor—is to treat the pneumonia with antibiotics and watch his hydration.

If he improves, we can do a few more things with the idea of making him more comfortable. We can drain the fluid from his lungs through a small catheter, rather than through a chest tube, which is a thumb-size tube placed between the ribs that can be uncomfortable. We would still pay particular attention to his comfort level, and if these smaller interventions caused him pain, we would give him morphine as needed.

If he were to stop breathing or if his heart were to stop beating, we would not resuscitate him. Resuscitation involves pumping on the chest and inserting a breathing tube in his mouth down into his lungs to pump oxygen in and out. It can also involve shocking him to try to restart his heart. We would instead let him go peacefully.

The third option is to give him pain medicine now and let nature takes its course. When he dies, we would not try to bring him back.

Since we are unable to ask Mr. Huzjak himself, we have to look to the family to decide what he would want in this situation.

Do you have any questions?

The family is silent.

I throw out another question. Is there anyone else that you would like me to talk to?

I have finished talking. The truth is on the table. Have my arguments pierced the wall of grief and denial?

Will the older sister break the silence, or will she defer to the brothers? I wait. I watch.

The older brother looks up from the floor and stares into my eyes directly, like a cop. "What's his condition?" he asks.

I am startled. Does he want a classification: grave, critical, stable, a one-word descriptor of the sort you see in a newspaper?

I realize I've fucked up. My presentation was too long and detailed. The basic information was lost and the larger questions missed.

"What about nutrition?" asks the younger brother even more aggressively.

What about it? I am taken aback by his tone. However, the man asked a question and he deserves an answer. Calmly, in a nonconfrontational way, I explain that we are concerned about nutrition, but the issues in order of urgency are his respiratory status and shortness of breath, his pneumonia, which can impair his respiratory status and his cardiovascular status.

I explain that his albumin, a marker of nutrition, is low. This is common in lung-cancer patients, but it isn't so low as to say that death from starvation is imminent, whereas death from these other problems is imminent.

So much for my hope of getting through to the Huzjaks. I am tired. I sense distrust not unlike the kind we had for doctors when I was growing up in black Detroit. I remind myself that in my state of mind I have no right to jump to conclusions. I haven't slept all night. My judgment may be intact, but my instincts are dulled. What should I have done differently?

Should I explain the word *imminent*? I ask myself. Is it too long? Am I being a tired asshole? I bite my tongue. Maybe this black doctor is resorting to classism to counteract racism, real or perceived. None of this is good.

The younger Huzjaks ask why their father is on a nasal cannula and not an oxygen mask. I explain that he has a kind of breathing problem called carbon dioxide retention that can be made worse if he is put on too much oxygen. His lungs are in such bad shape that he cannot get all the carbon dioxide out of his body, so his brain has become accustomed to high levels in his blood. The only reason he breathes is the brain stem's desire to get oxygen into his blood.

The wife of one of the brothers asks where I went to medical school. I recognize the question for what it is, a passive-aggressive way to avoid dealing with the problem.

I answer that I went to college and medical school at the University of Chicago. I let her know that others agree with me on what we are up against: a murderous disease that we can't slow down, let alone stop. We may be able to prolong Huzjak's misery, but at a cost of causing great pain. Claren has reviewed all the data, as have the doctors in the ER, as have the doctors on my team; there is universal agreement.

I have given them carefully reasoned, compassionate information and now list the white people who agree with me. The situation is absurd, and I know it in real time.

I wonder whether she knows that the University of Chicago is a good school. Nineteen eighty-six is just a few years after the *Bakke* decision, and talk of affirmative action is still ubiquitous in the news media. While it's tempting to ascribe the younger Huzjaks' distrust exclusively to racism, it may not be accurate.

I know that even when my white colleagues try to impress on the families of patients that the time has come to say good-bye, they run into resistance.

One brother asks what resuscitation is—like if his heart stops, or if he stops breathing. This is an appropriate question, perhaps even an opportunity to build understanding.

I describe resuscitation. I mention breathing for the patient with an Ambu bag and placing a tube down the throat into the lungs. I explain that a patient on a ventilator, with a tube in his throat, feels as if he is drowning, except that feeling goes on and on. I talk about chest compressions to get blood flowing if the heart stops. I describe electric shock.

Resuscitation is something I do well, maybe even get a thrill from. But I always got a nauseous feeling after a successful resuscitation. It is appropriate for a healthy person who has one problem causing the arrest.

If you restart the heart or restart the breathing, you buy time, fix the underlying problem, and the person ends up returning to life, perhaps even normal life. Unfortunately, in internal medicine, we do lots of resuscitations on patients who are destined to need it again in a few days and will continue needing it until they arrest and will not come back or until someone has an attack of common sense and says, "Enough!"

Huzjak's daughter begins to talk, saying that she speaks for her brothers. It's now obvious that she plays this role often. She wants everything done to save her father's life.

"Everything reasonable or everything possible?" I ask. I tell her that we feel that resuscitation is not reasonable in the event of cardiac or pulmonary arrest.

"Everything possible is everything reasonable, as far as we are concerned," she says.

As I walk to the residents' office, I feel sick to my stomach. I think about the younger Huzjaks. They will not feel the excruciating physical torture that being pulled from death will require. Their father will. They will not be performing these senseless acts of medical torture. I will. They will not be paying the bills. People paying higher health insurance rates will.

Economists have a name for this: "a moral hazard." A moral hazard occurs when a person making a decision is protected from its consequences.

Soon after meeting the Huzjaks, I sit down and, just for the hell of it, calculate how much useless, harmful care for this man could cost the system. I get to $250,000 just for the care we had provided and the care we are about to provide.

The number seems horrifying.

I am in the beginning of my career, and I believe that at some point problems of cost of care and elimination of useless, unscientific care would be solved either through controls by insurance companies or by the government declining to pay.

My prediction is wrong.

Now, three decades later, as I sit down with a pad of paper and start adding up expenses for a hypothetical patient similar to Huzjak, I realize that today he would probably receive a great deal more chemotherapy, perhaps well beyond the point where life extension or even delay in progression of disease are a possibility. The willingness of insurance companies to pay, and the willingness of private physicians to make a buck, have extended the standards of care enormously from three decades ago.

In addition, had he been brought into an ER in 2011, Huzjak would have been subjected to even greater abuse and an even larger number of obscenely expensive and ridiculous medical tests and procedures. There would definitely be more imaging—a magnetic-resonance-imaging study would be ordered to assess his brain damage. There would be CTs, lots of them. A CT in 1986 was a big deal. A patient stayed in the machine for more than an hour. Now, the rate-limiting step is how quickly your orderlies can get patients on and off the table. I can easily see the bill for a patient like Huzjak adding up to $600,000.

No one seems to argue with the estimate that about 24 percent of Medicare spending and about 15 percent of all health spending is incurred in the last year of a patient's life.

Why such a high proportion? Yes, a person whose body is failing is going to need a lot of medical care. Yet fleecing the system is in these numbers, too.

I have seen doctors do some horrible, irrational things under the guise of seeking to benefit patients. I have seen my colleagues disregard data in ways that ultimately benefit them financially: a bone marrow transplant for a breast-cancer patient, prophylactic doses of Aranesp and Procrit—these are only a few examples. The system rewards us for selling our goods and services, and we play the game.

However, I can't think of a single anecdote of doctors creating or encouraging situations where a patient who is ready to die is instead subjected to aggressive care. Even the greediest of doctors refrain from such behavior because they know that it's wrong. It's so wrong that you can't possibly justify it. Yet, patients demand this kind of care, and we oblige.

Americans don't understand death. We cannot accept that death will come, and thus we cannot make a plan, talk reasonably about it, work our way to understanding, to the basic part of our humanity. This attitude—a combination of perpetual optimism, refusing the dark, and not living in reality—is unfair to patients, doctors, and insurance companies.

AFTER receiving my marching orders from the younger Huzjaks, I search for explanations. Perhaps I care about Mr. Huzjak more than his flesh and blood. Perhaps they don't want to face other relatives who might blame them for having let old Huzjak die. Perhaps they don't understand the reality of their father's future. Perhaps they are unable to accept it. Perhaps I fucked up. Perhaps it's pigmentation. Perhaps it's class. My self-flagellation sets the stage for the torture I will have to inflict: this man will arrest and we will try to bring him back. He will experience the sensation of drowning as we intubate him and try to breathe for him. He will have pain and discomfort that I will not be able to control. No, let's call things by their proper name: he will have pain and discomfort, and I will exacerbate this with the pain and discomfort of futile treatment.

We aren't really trying to benefit Huzjak; we know we can't. Instead we do harm, because we are instructed to do so.

I tell the intern that Huzjak is a full code, that I failed to get a DNR or any limits on his care. If he has a cardiac or respiratory arrest, we are obligated to perform lifesaving measures. Whatever it takes. "We have to four-plus him," I say. It's the equivalent of saying 110 percent. We have to really try to resuscitate the guy, not just go through the motions. We have to be sincere in our efforts as we suspend disbelief.

As the internal-medicine doctor in charge, I am responsible for organizing the various consulting specialist teams and their access to the patient for treatment. In this case I am orchestrating a macabre dance, pretending to be saving a life that cannot be saved. The dance is grandiose. I tell the intern to call for a cardiac consult. Ask for an echo to see whether Huzjak has fluid around the heart. Call pulmonary and get a bronchoscopy—a scope will be threaded through Huzjak's nose or mouth and down into the lungs to look at the bronchial tubes. Pulmonary will look for obstructions and run cultures to determine what bug might be causing pneumonia.

Call thoracic surgery, too. We may need a "pericardial window" from the pericardial space to the peritoneal cavity. The goal would be to let the pericardial effusion drain from the space surrounding the heart—where it's interfering with heart function—into the abdomen.

We will definitely need to insert a chest tube and perform a procedure called sclerosis. We will place an irritating material—talc—in the pleural space to cause inflammation of the membranes. Inflammation will cause the membranes to stick together, thereby eliminating the pleural space in which fluids could accumulate.

I hope to God we don't have to perform a lung biopsy to see whether Huzjak has lymphangitic spread of his cancer, if the cancer has gotten into the tissue where air is transferred. If the answer is affirmative, this will only add another untreatable condition to the roster of untreatable, fatal conditions on this patient's chart.

First thing, get a CT of his head with and without contrast, if possible, but we have to get one without to clear his head for a lumbar puncture. ("Clear his head" was our language for making sure it was safe to do the lumbar puncture without danger of causing the patient's brainstem to herniate, which means to be sucked down the spine.) For an LP, we'll tap into his spine to collect a sample of cerebrospinal fluid for microbiological and cytological analysis.

An intern asks whether instead of the CT we want to do an eye exam to clear him for the LP. I say no, we will wait for the CT, even if that delays his workup a day or two. In the old days, residents were trained to look into the back of the eye with a funduscope, to look for evidence of intracranial pressure before the LP. We were taught to do that in case we had to do an emergent LP and could not get the patient to the CT quickly. But an eye exam isn't as accurate.

If you do an LP on a patient who has a tumor blocking the third ventricle of the brain, you can cause herniation of the brain. The brain swells and is forced down the top of the spinal canal. When this happens, the patient goes rigid, takes some deep breaths, and dies. In medicine, there are only a few sudden deaths, and this is one of them.

I could do it, I was good at it, but I was not going to attempt it with this patient. It wasn't worth the personal risk of being wrong. Huzjak is going to die, and if he dies during or after the LP, it will be attributed to the LP.

I don't want to be blamed for a death that is coming with or without the LP.

I push the intern to get these tests in quickly so she can get to her other patients, put them to bed, and get home to get some rest. Huzjak is one of about thirty patients for whom I am responsible. (As a resident, I am supervising two interns, each of whom has to take care of six to seventeen patients.) Huzjak is sucking up time, which means less attention to go around. As a result, hospital stays are prolonged. Patients can get sick from bugs they pick up in hospitals. They have to be treated, and some do poorly. These, too, are costs, and they have to be counted.

A patient's wife is pissed. We didn't answer all her questions about her husband's condition. She looks like a person who is used to getting her way, and in this case her sense of entitlement is justified.

Also, some poor guy didn't get the full attention his pain deserves, again because we were busy with Huzjak, the patient who cannot benefit from our care.

I pray for my patients, and that morning I pray that Huzjak is not really aware of what we are about to do to him.

Chapter 11

God Is Calling

AFTER THE LAB TESTS come back, we move on to thoracentesis. We do this for two reasons: to diagnose why the fluid has accumulated in Huzjak's chest to begin with, whether the effusion is caused by malignancy or an infection, and to treat the problem by draining the accumulated fluid, thereby giving the lungs the space they need to expand. Two students hold Huzjak in place as we seat him at the side of the bed. He flops forward with his arms over a dinner-tray stand (dinner-tray stands are for this procedure—you can adjust the height of the stand to each patient). Usually, a patient doesn't need to be held in place. Alas, Huzjak is unable to take directions and lacks control of his faculties.

Beth, the intern, percusses Huzjak's back with her fingers to find the area where the fluid is. She places the middle finger of one hand over the patient's back, then taps on it with three fingers of the other hand. When you get a hollow sound, you are over an area unencumbered by fluid. When you get a dull sound, you are over an effusion. (I use the same method to find two-by-fours beneath drywall when I do home repair projects.) Beth marks the dull-sounding area with a permanent marker. I follow behind her and confirm the spot. I ask her to feel the ribs and let me know where the needle should go in.

After that, Beth paints a six-inch, yellow rectangle with a topical antiseptic to create a sterile field, killing the bacteria on the skin before we start sticking needles into the pleural cavity. She stretches on a pair of surgical gloves. I open the thoracentesis kit. She takes the sterile paper drape, removes some paper covering sticky tape-like strips, and places the sheet over Huzjak's back.

A med student hands Beth a large sheet of paper with a three-inch-square hole. The area Beth had crisscrossed with a marker peeks through the hole in the sheet. Good sheet placement. Now comes the tricky part, something that scares interns: you have to stick the needle directly above the rib, as close to the top of the rib as you can. Go a bit higher and you will hit a nerve, an artery, and a vein.

Beth puts her instruments in order, checking them. She breaks a glass ampoule and sucks up lidocaine, a topical anaesthetic, into a syringe. She places a small, 23-gauge needle on the syringe and looks to me for approval.

I prefer hitting the bone with the needle first. Then I raise the needle a tad, still keeping the tip in the skin, to clear the bone. First, you squeeze out a squirt of lidocaine, creating a small bleb in the skin, something akin to a mosquito sting. Then you pull back the needle, to make sure you aren't aspirating blood. If you don't see blood, you keep pushing forward. You keep moving, paving the way with lidocaine, and you do this until you start aspirating straw-colored fluid.

I give her the go-ahead. She sticks the thin needle into Huzjak's skin at the site of the mark. He screams, but doesn't move. She is visibly upset. I reassure her, and she finishes injecting the numbing medicine under the skin.

Beth knows the procedure well and executes it perfectly. She presses into the back slowly and lets me know when she feels the needle passing just over the top of the rib. Huzjak screams again, this time even louder.

When we see the fluid, Beth pulls out the 23-gauge needle and inserts a larger, 16-gauge needle into the numbed area. She pulls back the piston and the syringe fills with fluid. Even in this situation, it's satisfying to see procedures work out exactly as they should.

She fills the syringe, turns off a valve at the top of the needle, unscrews the syringe, and hands it to the med students, whose job is to take the fluid to the labs that will analyze the chemistry, cytology, and cell count. She places a larger syringe on the needle and slowly pulls up the fluid, 100 cc of it. Now we are just draining the fluids. We repeat this operation fifteen times, draining a liter and a half. This takes about forty minutes. If you do it too fast, the patient will lose blood pressure.

These invasive procedures are just the beginning. We will be back, almost certainly. We might be performing sclerosis, to eliminate the pleural cavity, or we might be putting in the chest tube.

Beth and I prepare tubes of the fluid for the labs. They will analyze it for chemistries, gram stain it for bacteria, and culture it for bacteria and tuberculosis. The big bag—over a liter—goes to cytology. They will spin it down and look for sediment, which I am sure has cancer in it.

I remind Beth to order a portable chest X-ray to make sure that we didn't poke a hole in the lung. An air leak can cause a pneumothorax. In a severe case, a collapsed lung can be deadly.

DAVE Johnson, the pulmonary fellow, comes by. He has a reputation for being a "have scope, will travel" kind of guy—he will scope anything for the weakest of reasons. He *wants* to bronch poor Huzjak. He is so eager to do the procedure, he doesn't even bother to examine the patient.

I am pissed at his enthusiasm, but part of "doing everything" is to see if the bronchus is obstructed and needs to be opened up with radiation or by burning a hole with the hospital's new laser.

More than anything, I need a brushing of the bronchial tree for culture. Maybe we can find a bacterial infection we can treat. I doubt that will wake Huzjak up and improve his quality of life, but there is a chance. Alternatively, the bronch findings could be so bad that they will make his family do the right thing.

Wild Dave schedules the scoping for first thing the next morning. I have to downright argue with him to wait till the workup is complete. I want to wait in part because I want to see what the CT shows and in part because I keep hoping that the younger Huzjaks will come to their senses and realize that their father doesn't need to be bronched.

The procedure Dave is wild about has two potential downsides. The scope will obstruct Huzjak's already compromised oxygenation, which could cause arrhythmia or even a heart attack. If either occurs, we will have to put him on a ventilator. And if the scope punctures one of the

many funguslike tumors that are surely surrounding Huzjak's bronchial tubes, he will likely drown in his own blood.

Wild Dave relents, agreeing to hold off for a day or so, until I get a
CT of the chest.

NEXT, I have to deal with the thoracic surgery resident, Steve Edge. He is
much more reasonable. At first he is pissed at me for calling and bothering
them with a request to work on someone who clearly needs a priest to give
him last rites instead of a thoracic surgeon to crack his chest open. I am
delighted that he is pissed. It is a pleasure to find a surgeon with good
clinical judgment, a surgeon not eager to cut. Once he reads the chart and
understands the situation, he offers to talk to the family and hang black
crepe.

I tell him that many of us have already tried.

A CT of Huzjak's head had been ordered by the ER. Now, only a day
later, the radiologist has read it. There is no evidence of metastases on the
noncontrasted scan. The third ventricle is open okay to do an LP. We are
unable to get a CT with contrast. We cannot exclude a brain met without
contrast, but I am not thrilled with giving the poor guy contrast anyway.
His serum creatinine of 1.7 tells me that he is dry and needs watering.
Under these conditions, contrast can lead to renal failure. We'll get the
contrast test later.

I work with a third-year medical student and give Huzjak an LP. Yet
Huzjak continues to respond to one thing only: pain. He opens his eyes,
grunts, and screams, when presented with noxious stimuli. The third-
year is uncomfortable with having to cause pain for no reason. He says
he feels like this human is being treated like a lab animal.

To this day, I think about poor Huzjak screaming and moaning as
we position him and stick the needles in his back. I wonder whether this
and similar experiences as a doc gave me post-traumatic stress disorder
for which I have never been treated. I mean this literally. We cause pain
to our patients, and often they die no matter what we do. One proven
way to avoid feelings of loss is to dull all feelings, to detach. If you become emotionally involved, you become ineffective. And if you don't
become friendly with your patients, it's a whole lot easier when they die.

Many of my colleagues have learned to ward off PTSD by becoming assholes. This coping mechanism wasn't right for me, but I have developed others. To distract myself from the clinic, I venture into politics and highly technical areas, such as cancer screening. Numbers signifying "survival" and "cause-specific mortality" are so much easier to accept than the death and suffering they codify.

I review Huzjak's lab tests, looking for an easy root cause for his being obtunded. I review his metabolites, I look at his thyroid function, I look at all the blood gases. I look at the CT scan of his head.

We would later perform a CT of the head with contrast and a CT of the chest. His spinal-fluid cytology comes back negative for tumor. At first I am relieved that he doesn't have evidence of carcinomatous meningitis, tumor cells scattered all over his brain, and then I realize that the standard for ruling out carcinomatous meningitis is three negative LPs. Should we do two more of these?

Around 5:00 p.m., Beth, Claren, and I see Huzjak. Claren hears our verbal report and thumbs through the chart. As he examines Huzjak, the daughter walks in. Claren greets her and suggests that we all talk.

Beth quickly finds a room down the hall for some privacy. Claren is masterful and polite as he explains that Huzjak is dying of his lung cancer, and the process can be long. He describes what we are doing and suggests that it might be more appropriate to focus our efforts on keeping him comfortable. He notes that the only response we have gotten from him is expressions of pain when we move him or subject him to procedures.

She reiterates her desire that everything be done. Claren asks whether she means that she wants us to do everything reasonable to keep him comfortable. No, she says, that's not what the family wants. We are to treat all illnesses.

The next day, the CT of the chest shows the extent of Huzjak's tumor bilaterally. There's lots of it and with lymphangitic spread. The air exchange surfaces are thickened by tumor.

Still, we are in a chicken-and-egg situation. Does the pneumonia cause him to be obtunded or does obtundation lead to the pneumonia? We see disease in the liver. There is still some pleural effusion, some pericardial effusion.

At this point, Wild Dave Johnson takes Huzjak to the bronch suite and, with his resident, bronchs him. I send the students so they can watch. Someone should witness this travesty. Later, they tell me that Johnson used no anaesthesia. He was concerned that pain control could cause Huzjak to stop breathing.

They go through the nose, passing the throat, into the larynx, and on into the bronchus. They examine both sides, seeing tumor in the bronchial tubes—roughened, yellowish-red surfaces in the bronchial tubes on both sides, extensive cancer involving both lungs. They see near-obstruction and pus in the left main-stem bronchus and get a sample for culture. This means it's likely a postobstructive pneumonia; things that are blocked or partially blocked get infected. The bronch also produces pictures of the partially obstructed bronchus with pus and pictures of the cancer in the bronchial tubes.

Wild Dave withdraws the scope and observes Huzjak for an hour to make sure he is okay. Even he realizes that old men don't take trauma like this well. He returns the patient to the room and leaves a note with pictures.

Huzjak stays in the hospital for the next three days. He is quietly there, out of everyone's way. The nurses turn him frequently, to keep him from getting bedsores. His blood cultures grow gram positive cocci, a bug sensitive to ampicillin and gentamicin.

He is surviving and seems to be doing well, except he is not waking up. He is not running a fever, but he may still have bugs the antibiotics haven't killed. And slowly but steadily he is losing blood pressure.

We have to worry about nutrition. I have Beth pass a Dobhoff tube into him. This thin tube with a weight at the bottom goes up the nose and down through the throat, esophagus, and stomach, stopping in the first part of the small bowel. The nurses hang a bag of white, milky-looking nutrients and drip in twelve hundred calories a day. This provides some nutrition and some hydration.

Eventually, we convert his IV to a central line. We place it in the subclavian vein, another procedure for Beth and one of the students. The X-ray shows no damage to the lung and perfect positioning of the catheter near the atrium of the heart. The X-ray also shows pneumonia. It could have been there all along, when he was dry. Now that he has been hydrated, or, as we say in the language of distancing, "watered," wet bacteria and wet pus have been rendered visible.

APART from procedures, Huzjak requires less and less attention. We check his labs daily, but he becomes a nursing problem, not a doctor's problem. The nurses complain a bit, asking about *placement*. The phrase means they think he should be discharged to a nursing home or a hospice.

Yet, Huzjak remains in the hospital. He needs to be on antibiotics for two weeks without running a fever before the meds going into his central line can be stopped.

After he has been in the hospital for nearly three weeks, Claren calls a family meeting. I see another desperate attempt to make the younger Huzjaks come to their senses.

This time Claren brings in another doctor, someone white, with a blue-collar upbringing—David Ginn. Ginn comes from a long line of white Arkansas sharecroppers. His father is an auto mechanic. Ginn is tall, lanky, crusty, sometimes macabre, the sort of guy who finds it an ordeal to wear a tie.

As Ginn comes over to provide a second opinion, I sit in with the interns and students. Claren introduces us all to the family and once more explains what's happening to Huzjak, with the latest updates and information we have. He says that we need to talk about limitations of care and asks Ginn for his thoughts.

"I've seen Mr. Huzjak's X-rays and labs, and I've examined him," Ginn begins. He knows what he is up against, so he puts on a performance. He comes up to an X-ray view box and turns it on.

First, he puts on a bone scan. "This is a normal bone scan." He leaves it in place and puts on another bone scan. "And this is your father's bone scan." The difference is obvious. Huzjak's scan is shocking, lit up with metastases. "It ain't normal."

Ginn takes down the scans and clips a chest X-ray onto the light box. "This is a normal chest X-ray." He places another X-ray next to it. "And this is your father's chest X-ray. It ain't normal."

He keeps going. "This is a normal liver on CT scan, and this is your father's CT. It ain't normal." Next, he does the same for bronchoscopy. "The red and irregular yellow areas are cancer," he points out. "Your father has a disease that medical science cannot treat. He has widely metastatic, widely spread lung cancer. There are no good treatments, and he has had the only reasonable treatment, which is not very good, and it did not help him."

Ginn is readying for the finale, and it's a good one:

"God is calling, and who are we to say no?"

The family doesn't budge.

ON my last day on service, Huzjak spikes a fever to 103°. We examine him, culture his blood and urine, and get a portable chest X-ray. We can't find a reason for the fever. We call the daughter to report the change in status.

Over the next several hours we change his antibiotics to ceftazidime and clindamycin in an effort to cover what we might be missing. He has some diarrhea, likely due to the tube feeding. We send it off for study. Pseudomembranous colitis caused by *C. difficile* growing as a result of the antibiotics could explain the fever.

His respiratory rate and heart rate increase suddenly. The blood pressure starts to drop. I hate using ICU beds for someone who is dying anyway, but I have no choice. The ICU is in the building next door. Huzjak is wheeled over by Beth and the two students, with two nurses from the floor. The daughter and a son walk along.

Huzjak stabilizes in the ICU. Ironically, I get transferred to ICU the same night, replacing the resident who checked Huzjak in. We have fourteen beds, and nine of them are occupied. We have some sick people in the unit. Four are on ventilators and six are on pressors. Pressors are medicines such as dopamine or Levophed, given intravenously to keep a patient's blood pressure consistent with life. We have people with infections, people with respiratory issues, especially COPD bronchitis, and emphysema. The worst is a twenty-four-year-old girl with herpes meningitis.

The next morning, I realize that I am weirdly delighted to find Huz-jak alive. Perhaps it's because he has turned into a fixture in my life. I worry about him often, realizing how close he is to death to begin with, worrying even more about bringing him to its brink. Yet here he is still, resilient, surviving.

He hasn't changed much since I sent him to the unit. He actually seems more comfortable, or maybe more obtunded. Whatever the reason, he seems to be in less discomfort.

His family is keeping a vigil. In the old days, I would only see the daughter. Now I also see her brothers, their wives, even some grandkids. I greet them, but they are guarded, minimally polite.

I do my work on all the patients and get three new admissions. As we are working up new admits, the nurse responsible for Huzjak quietly asks me to come over. He is throwing a lot of ectopic, abnormal heart-beats. His blood pressure is lower than it was last time we measured it. I ask for an EKG and go on to care for the other patients.

The EKG shows the extra abnormal beats, but also shows T waves across the anterior of the heart. I was taught to call this pattern the tomb-stone Ts—they indicate a myocardial infarction. He is having a heart attack, likely a big one, and there isn't a thing we can do to slow it down.

Drugs aren't an option. We just got clot-busting drugs in the past year, but a metastatic cancer patient is not a candidate. These drugs are more likely to kill him than help him.

I call Claren and ask what he would like me to do.

"Let it evolve if necessary," he says. "Give him some nitroglycerin if his blood pressure will allow it." I dare to give Huzjak a couple of inches of nitropaste to the skin. We can wipe it off if his already low blood pressure becomes a problem.

After three hours, at almost exactly midnight, he develops bradycar-dia, a slow heart rate of about thirty. He almost certainly has infarcted part of the Purkinje system, a group of nerve fibers in the heart that regulates heart rate. His blood pressure is dropping, too.

The nurses usher his son out. I get the endotracheal cart open as a nurse breaths for him with an Ambu bag. The intern notes that his pulse is only thirty to forty per minute. I open his mouth and slide a light and a blade into his mouth. I see the vocal cords and slide an endotracheal tube into his trachea. I inflate the balloon that holds it in place and connect the Ambu bag. We continue to breathe for him as Sarah, the ICU intern, listens to his lungs for breath sounds. The next few seconds are tense.

"Yes." Sarah nods. This means I had placed the tube into the lungs and not into the esophagus. With some relief, I listen to assure myself that I got the tube in the right place. I even listen over his stomach, to make sure I am not pumping air into his stomach instead of his lungs.

Next, we quickly put a wire through his triple lumen. We use a wire with a catheter capable of pacing his heart. We use this to stimulate his heart to beat at eighty beats per minute. His blood pressure is still eighty systolic, which is low. As it starts to go lower, I order a dopamine drip to support his blood pressure.

We seem to have taken over his entire body, taking control of all of its functions. Chest compression is the only procedure left that we had not yet done. I wonder if I will have the guts to order the nurses and interns to pump on this guy's chest in a code, and Huzjak is considerate enough not to put me in that position.

His body temperature at night swings from fever at 103°, to cold at 96°. We conclude that he has also had an infarct in his thalamus, a part of the brain that controls the body temperature. The nurses put a water blanket on him. To even out his body temperature, we circulate water of whatever temperature we see fit. We give him a diuretic when we decide that it's time for him to pee.

By 6:00 a.m. I am sitting at the foot of Huzjak's bed. I feel like shit about all the pain I caused while using his body to teach LPs, central lines, and thoracentesis to the interns and medical students. Here he is, the guy whose family frustrated the hell out of me. He is just lying here quietly. I know that he is trying to die, and his family and the rest of us won't let him.

I sit there with him on a ventilator, with a pacer, on pressors, under a temperature blanket. This black kid from Detroit whose credentials, competence, and education the Huzjak family has questioned can now decide his vital signs for the day. I can set his respiratory rate and his respiratory volume. Also, his heart rate, blood pressure, and body temperature.

Around 8:00 a.m. the next morning, Huzjak goes into ventricular fibrillation and loses his blood pressure, possibly due to another heart attack. We usher out his family—his daughter, a son, and a grandchild.

Six or seven of us are in the room—doctors, nurses, students. There is nothing to do, so we stand somberly, silently, with our heads down, some of us praying, others tearing up watching him go into cardiac arrest. It would have been so much more humane if the Huzjaks had been there instead of us, but that was the choice they made.

We turn the blower and the pacer off and tell the family that we are sorry, but Mr. Huzjak died at 8:20 a.m. "We were unable to resuscitate him from the second heart attack," we tell them.

They take it well.

I call Claren and let him know that it's finally over. He expresses his gratitude to the interns, nurses—and me. He asks how I'm feeling. A decent guy, he knows how difficult "saving" Huzjak was.

PART III

More Is Better

Chapter 12

Ole Boys' Club

BY THE MIDDLE of my second year of residency I realize that I want to be in a subspecialty where I will be working with patients who are genuinely and demonstrably ill. In October 1986, I call John Ultmann, a professor and friend at the University of Chicago.

"Dr. Ultmann, I have been thinking about what I want to do in medicine, and I want to do oncology."

"Ott-i-ss," says Ultmann with the Austrian accent that is remarkably thick for someone who came to New York at age thirteen. "I have been waiting for this call."

ULTMANN had a deeper appreciation of ethics—and failure thereof—than your average doctor. Born in Vienna in 1925, he deeply understood the power of a bad idea. He watched fascism take root in the city of his birth, and it was about him. The ideology was built on the idea that people like John—the Jews—were not fully human.

His understanding of cancer was deeply rooted, too. His mother died of it when he was ten.

After graduating from the Bronx High School of Science, Ultmann returned to Europe wearing a GI's uniform. He fought in Italy, then returned to Austria, where his job was to identify and interrogate Nazi criminals and gather information for the war-crimes trials at Nuremberg. He attended Brooklyn and Oberlin Colleges and then the College of Physicians and Surgeons at Columbia University.

He became interested in cancer while working at New York City hospitals. As the field of oncology came into existence in 1973, Ultmann was one of its founders. He was a coauthor of the specialty's first-ever board-certification exam.

Ultmann had a rectangular face (wide jowls, a square shock of hair). His speech was precise, Teutonic, his manners courtly. I met him during my second year of med school, during the first day of his legendary pathophysiology class. Ultmann's research was in lymphoma, a cancer of the immune system that would ultimately kill him. His other interest was politics. You could argue that the two interests were inextricable from each other.

Lymphoma was particularly important politically: it was a battlefield where the government-funded war on cancer was scoring a victory. Many forms of lymphoma lend themselves to treatment. Massive tumors can literally melt away, and in some cases patients get long-term responses, even cures.

An enormous amount of research money was being pumped into the field. Grand promises were being made, and victories were needed to allow the establishment to perpetuate the claim that the cure was around the corner.

Ultmann could spend the morning making rounds at UChicago and late afternoons behind closed doors on Capitol Hill or on the NIH campus in Bethesda, Maryland, cutting deals in rooms that were still filled with smoke, lobbying for money for the cancer program, helping shape the scientific agenda of the National Cancer Institute, kissing the hands of the right grandes dames, flattering the needed politicos, getting drug companies to write the right checks—and unabashedly taking a cut for the University of Chicago.

THE University of Chicago was—and still is—the kind of place that makes the extraordinary seem ordinary. When I was there, one could become blasé about seeing a Nobel laureate on the quad. Sightings of the writer Saul Bellow, economist Milton Friedman, physician Charles Huggins, or geneticist George Beadle were almost everyday occurrences.

Huggins liked to hang out with students, introducing himself as "the

SOB who won a Nobel Prize for cutting off a poor bastard's balls."
Huggins, who was eighty when I met him, won the 1966 prize for
physiology or medicine for discovering that an endocrine disruption
could be used to control the spread of malignancy. This was more than
cutting off balls: it was a new paradigm in cancer treatment.

When I was an undergraduate living in a dorm called Burton-Judson
Courts, George Stigler, an economist who would win a Nobel Prize in
1982, was one of our dorm fellows. Basically, this meant that he hung
out and ate lunch with the undergraduates. At one point, he and I debated the US government's bailout of Chrysler. Stigler thought it was
wrongheaded to protect a company that was unable to function on its
own. I thought it was essential because I knew a bunch of people who
worked on the Chrysler assembly line, and the prospect of their being
out of work struck me as unacceptable. This was an interesting friendship: a free-market economist and future Nobel Prize winner and a kid
from Burlingame Street, struggling to preserve his footing in two
worlds.

Another acquaintance, Leon Jacobson, was one of the first doctors to
use chemotherapy successfully. He used nitrogen mustard, a derivative
of a World War I poison gas, to treat leukemia and lymphoma. He was
also the discoverer of something he called erythroprotein, a hormone
that induced the body to produce hemoglobin. Later, the protein would
be renamed erythropoietin. Jacobson also discovered the basis for bone
marrow transplants—and he served as chief physician of the Manhattan
Project.

At the University of Chicago you could take a course taught by Arthur Rubenstein, an endocrinologist, who discovered how to measure
insulin in the blood; or Arthur Herbst, who linked clear cell cancer of
the vagina to DES (diethylstibestrol, a synthetic estrogen); or Seymour
Glagov, who linked cholesterol to heart disease; or Donald F. Steiner, who
discovered the precursor of insulin and how the human body synthesizes
insulin; or Elwood Jensen, who pioneered studies of the estrogen receptor; or Janet Rowley, who showed that a transposition of chromosomes
could produce a form of leukemia; or Janet's husband, Donald Rowley,
who invented the saltwater gelatin that is used on an EKG.

* * *

NATURALLY, Ultmann's pathophysiology class focused on lymphoma. As a scientist and a clinician, Ultmann saw lymphoma as a set of distinct diseases that each carried different risks. He showed that therapy had to be determined based on disease type and its stage. Treatment had to be interdisciplinary, combining chemo, radiation, and surgery, and the only way to find out what worked was through rigorously designed clinical experiments, where one group gets Treatment A and another gets Treatment B.

After class, I came up to Ultmann to ask a question, and we ended up talking for about fifteen minutes.

"Ott-i-ss, I can already tell you are going to become an oncologist," Ultmann said, concluding that conversation.

This was the beginning of a friendship. It was obvious from the start that we understood each other's origin. He was a refugee, as, in a sense, was I. Affirmative action gave me the opportunity to become a doctor. He attended school courtesy of the GI Bill. With his goodwill, Herr Doktor Ultmann let me know that he understood where I came from and what I had to do to survive.

During my third year of med school, I was assigned to him for an internal-medicine rotation. Ultmann was like no other attending I ever saw. His formality was extreme, aggressive. You presented the patient to him in front of the patient, at the bedside, without notes: "Dr. Ultmann, this is Mrs. So-and-So. Mrs. So-and-So is fifty-five years old. She comes to us with the chief complaint . . ." You had to do all that knowing that Ultmann would crush you verbally if he detected imprecision.

He either liked you or didn't like you. If he didn't like you, it was because you weren't trying. Tardiness was not tolerated. Neither was frivolity of any sort. Both connoted disrespect.

Once, a resident put a smiley face on a patient's record, causing Ultmann to go bananas: "This is a legal record, this is an official record, how dare she desecrate the record!" To him, desecration of a record was a form of denial of humanity. He was not just treating cancer. He was trying to eradicate lies, complacency, and disrespect.

His rules were straightforward: You don't deviate from the science. You don't make it up as you are going along. You have to have a reason to give the drugs you are giving. You have to be able to quote literature that supports what you are doing. You have to tell patients the truth.

His moral principles, to me, were jesuitical.

WHEN I call him from Case Western to say that I am ready to go into oncology, Ultmann shifts into Socratic questioning of my motivations. It's not enough that I am going into oncology per his prediction. I have to go into oncology *for the right reasons.*

"Ott-i-ss, why do you want to do oncology?"

"Oncology has the right mix of science, medicine, and public policy."

Most people in high school thought that I would become a lawyer and a politician. Though I am going into medicine, in oncology, I will have the opportunity to use my God-given gift of speech. As an oncopolitician, Ultmann appreciates this.

That oncologists make decent money also influenced me. I prefer to give money as little thought as possible, but at that time I was deep in debt. I wouldn't pay off med school bills until age forty-three.

"We want you to apply to Stanford, UCSF, University of Chicago, Memorial Sloan-Kettering Cancer Center, Dana-Farber, Mass General, University of Pennsylvania, Johns Hopkins, and the National Cancer Institute." *We* is Herr Doktor Ultmann, a royal *we.* "You will get a letter of recommendation from us. You will keep detailed notes. Every time you see a place, you will rank every one of them until that point. Then you will call and tell us what your choice is."

That Ultmann writes my first recommendation likely determines the seriousness with which my fellowship application is taken at every one of these places. I meet with the director of each of these top institutions, and the choice seems clearly mine to make. When I return to Case Western, I call Ultmann.

"Dr. Ultmann, my first choice is Memorial Sloan-Kettering." It's an understandable choice. Memorial is a venerable academic institution. Just being considered for a fellowship there is an honor. Training at Memorial opens doors.

If the silence on the other end is an indication, Ultmann disagrees. I can see that I have made a mistake.

"If you go to Memorial, we will never speak with you again," he says finally.

"But, Dr. Ultmann, that was one of the places you wanted me to interview."

"Precisely. We wanted you to *interview* there. We didn't want you to *go* there."

"In that case, my first choice is the National Cancer Institute," I say, regrouping.

Suddenly I can see what Ultmann is thinking. Memorial is the place to learn to become a consummate clinical oncologist. NCI is the place to become a researcher. This has to be determined by his view of my strengths and weaknesses, his vision for my career. Perhaps he would have chosen Memorial for another of his protégés.

NCI is undeniably the place where the specialty of medical oncology had been invented in the 1950s and 1960s. In 1988, it was still the headquarters of the war on cancer, the place where bold strategies were being forged and where new drugs were being developed, the place where the cures would come from. At Case Western, I heard Emil Frei, a former NCI researcher, give a talk titled "How I Cured Childhood Leukemia." And he had, together with colleague Emil Freireich. (Along the way, this duo of physician-scientists erected articles of faith that would guide oncology for over half a century.)

Vincent DeVita, the NCI director and a friend of Ultmann's, was also one of the developers of the MOPP regimen for the treatment of Hodgkin's lymphoma. MOPP is a four-drug combination chemotherapy regimen consisting of the drugs mustargen, oncovin, procarbazine, and prednisone, which was developed for the treatment of Hodgkin's Lymphoma. NCI breast cancer researcher Mark Lippman did original work on blocking estrogen receptors in breast cancers.

The institute's influence extended into academia, too. It funded cancer centers as well as groups of physicians who banded together into "cooperative groups" to conduct clinical trials. Since the field of medical oncology was invented at NCI, all institutions that developed cancer programs by necessity had to hire people who had trained at NCI. More than half of the NCI-designated cancer centers were run by people who had trained at the institute. Former fellows ran the cooperative groups, too.

The institute controlled the purse strings for basic and clinical cancer research done in the United States. Some of this research was transforming medical practice. For example, the Pittsburgh-based cooperative group called the National Surgical Adjuvant Breast and Bowel Project had caused surgeons to abandon the brutal Halsted mastectomy in favor of conservative procedures followed by radiation.

Even outside oncology, NCI's impact was massive. In the 1950s, NCI pathologist Alan Rabson showed that the herpes virus hides in nerves, then comes to the surface in skin eruptions. In 1988, I knew that NCI retrovirus researcher Robert Gallo had discovered the HTLV-3 virus that caused AIDS. Later, the virus would be called HIV.

The institute's fellowship program was unique. A standard fellowship lasted two years and was entirely about clinical work. The NCI fellowship consisted of a year in the clinic, followed by two years of research, which could be anything from heavy-duty bench science to number-crunching in epidemiology and biostatistics.

"Where will you be tomorrow afternoon?" Ultmann asks, concluding our telephone conversation.

"I will be doing intensive care rotation at the VA."

"What's the number there?"

A day goes by. I am resuscitating a lung-cancer patient. A secretary—a black woman with a Southern accent—interrupts me to say, "There is a Dr. Broder from the National Cancer Institute who wants to talk with you."

"You'll have to take a message," I say, returning to the grim, futile business.

After it ends—the patient dies—I call and get patched through to Broder, director of the NCI Clinical Oncology Program.

"Dr. Brawley," says the voice on the line. I had met Broder at the interview, and he looked as if he could go from morose to Groucho Marx funny in the space of one sentence. "I have been instructed to offer you a job."

After accepting the job, I call Ultmann. The pronouncement I hear over the phone will guide my career:

"Ott-i-ss . . . Now you know that oncology is an ole boys' club. You are now part of that ole boys' club, and your job—and your payback—is to get as many blacks and women into the club as you can."

Chapter 13

Snuffy's War

ON JULY 1, 1988, when I showed up on the NIH campus as a new fellow at the NCI and a fresh conscript in the War on Cancer, I believed that the cure was just around the corner. The war rhetoric was in the air. Not knowing what we didn't know, many of us believed that the cure could emerge in any clinical trial. A genuine war was being fought, directed by aggressive generals.

This was a medical war of unprecedented proportions. Until the War on Cancer, progress in medicine was usually haphazard. Insights could be generated by individual scientists working at the bench. Treatments were proposed, tested, rejected. Some—such as the Halsted mastectomy—lingered too long out of deference to esteemed professors who championed them.

Cancer would be different. Here, a core strategy was being executed through a coordinated, generously funded National Cancer Program. This strategic approach promised to produce a specialty rooted in evidence rather than trial and error and the tyranny of scientific potentates. The emerging treatments for cancer would be grounded in clinical evidence and reason. A rational basis would mean that medical decisions in oncology would be straightforward.

I had some understanding of the weapons we were using to defeat cancer. Our chemotherapy drugs seemed good. It seemed logical that more drug would have a greater effect than less drug. Anyone who died of cancer died because they didn't get enough chemo. Doctors at NCI were experimenting with heroic doses of chemotherapy and *dose intensity* was the most important piece of the jargon of the era. Finding dose-limiting toxicities and kicking them out of the way was the name of the game. No one thought twice before taking a patient to the threshold of death and "rescuing" him at the last possible moment.

Massive doses of cytotoxic chemotherapy could destroy bone marrow. However, harvesting bone marrow before the start of treatment and reintroducing it after infusing massive doses of drugs would make it possible to cure cancer and let the patient recuperate.

Biological therapy seemed even more promising than chemo. I believed that we would soon develop the ability to mobilize the body's own power to fight cancer. The immune system would be trained to home in on rogue cells and, with precision, eradicate the disease. The year 2000 seemed to be a realistic target for finding the cure.

I felt as if I were a GI shipping out to Europe in the final months of the war, just before the Battle of the Bulge. There would be a few big battles and a lot of mopping up.

What would I do after victory? I had a plan: after completing the NCI fellowship, I would apply for a White House fellowship that would allow me to combine medicine with policy.

Imagine the challenges that would emerge after the cures were found. We would have to decide who got the cures first and how quickly. How would income, race, age, the severity of sickness, and the chances of cure figure into the formula for distribution of cures? Would a less sick prominent person get the cure before a sicker obscure person? In terms of resources involved and significance for mankind, the postcure era of cancer treatment would dwarf the task of reconstructing Europe under the Marshall Plan.

As I look at it now, I see that the declaration of the War on Cancer had more in common with the Spanish-American War than with World War II. The Spanish-American War started with mass hysteria whipped up by newspaper barons William Randolph Hearst and Joseph Pulitzer. The War on Cancer was waged in response to a public relations campaign orchestrated by the socialite Mary Lasker and her powerful friends in academia, business, and politics.

Mary, a woman with big hair and big plans, was the widow of Albert Lasker, one of the founders of the modern PR industry. She had an excellent operational plan for swaying the public agenda on cancer. She started by organizing an unofficial committee called the Panel of Consultants on the Conquest of Cancer to give the goal the sense of urgency and the appearance of consensus among key leaders.

This unofficial committee hammered the point that the cancer cure was in sight and could be achievable by the 1976 bicentennial of the United States. This seems absurd now, and—to many—it seemed utterly absurd then.

In 1971, Lasker's campaign reached its ultimate goal: President Richard Nixon signed the National Cancer Act, a law that made the War on Cancer a presidential priority. The act created a strong, politically influenced fiefdom within the National Institutes of Health. Unlike scientists who head the NIH who focused on arthritis, aging, dentistry, or mental disease, the director of the NCI is appointed by the president. The president also influences the institute by appointing members of the cancer institute's two principal advisory boards. One of these groups—the National Cancer Advisory Board—reviews all of the institute's scientific programs. Another—the President's Cancer Panel—is intended to inform the president about obstacles to the cure.

Originally, the latter panel included captains of industry—Benno Schmidt, a financier credited with coining the term *venture capital*, and Armand Hammer, chairman and CEO of Occidental Petroleum. Both of these men could call the president and get through. At one point, the National Cancer Advisory Board also included the much-trusted advice columnist Ann Landers.

Every year, the NCI director submits a Bypass Budget directly to the president. The word *bypass* refers to the director's ability to pass over the NIH and the Department of Health and Human Services hierarchy and inform the president how much money is needed to prosecute the War on Cancer. The Bypass Budget is largely ignored by policy makers, but it remains a quirky reminder of the specialness of the cancer program.

All of this may sound bureaucratic. But to us, the grunts in the War on Cancer, these special authorities translated into a sense of empowerment.

Another quirk of the war was more tangible: in recent years, the NCI directors have been the highest-paid presidential appointees, earning higher salaries than the vice president of the United States. This special status—and the boosts in appropriations that accompanied it—created a pressure on NCI directors to overstate the significance of their victories and, repeatedly, to promise the cure.

MY NCI fellowship begins with an administrative mistake. The orientation packet I receive at a morning meeting instructs me to report to an off-campus office building. I get on a shuttle bus—a big, dark blue GMC with government plates—and with a few minutes to spare arrive at an office building way out in northern Bethesda.

I can't spot any other fellows there. I try to find the office where the NCI meet-and-greet will take place, but no one seems to be able to help me. After brief, panicked searching, I borrow somebody's phone and dial the fellowship office, only to learn that at this exact time I am expected on the thirteenth floor of Building 10, the Clinical Center, at the heart of the NIH campus. Some numskull has screwed up my itinerary.

I catch the shuttle back and, feeling like crap, join the meeting about an hour and a half late. The two attending physicians at the front of the room are not about to let me slip in unnoticed.

"Dr. Brawley, you had one thing to do right today, and you didn't do it," says one of the two. "You didn't show up on time." I don't want to apologize or explain. The best I can do is bite my lip and mutter, "So this is my welcome."

As we start the rounds at the Clinical Center on my first day as a fellow, I notice its peculiar smell. It's partly a food scent, partly the smell of the building itself. The Clinical Center opened in 1953, and from the outside it looks something like public housing projects in New York or

Chicago. The place was outmoded by the seventies, but is still very much in use in the late eighties and beyond.

The clinical center doesn't have an emergency room, and it's not a hospital. Rather, it is the place where all of the major NIH conduct clinical research. The patients' rooms are positioned alongside a hallway in the front of the hospital, the laboratories alongside a parallel hallway in the back. This allows you to navigate between bench and bedside. NCI's medicine branch has the twelfth and thirteenth floors, sharing a part of the thirteenth floor with the pediatric oncology branch. The NCI surgery branch has the second floor.

I realize quickly that the place is ruled by warlords. Some of these men—they are all men—see no reason to control their tempers. One of my supervisors demonstrates displeasure by smashing a chair against a wall. We fellows take solace in the fact that he didn't hit anybody. Clashes between the department directors could get nasty fast, and their affairs—with secretaries and nurses—are brazenly conducted in plain sight.

IN the mid-1980s, NCI is not exclusively about cancer. Several of our labs are also trying to find the cure for the rapidly spreading immune deficiency illness, and the Clinical Center is filling with dying young men. NCI has a large supply of pharmaceutical compounds and an expertise in evaluating them for activity. Indeed, AIDS—as the disease later came to be known—often sparks malignancies, particularly lymphoma and Kaposi's sarcoma.

Researchers at the institute ponder the immune system and the role of retroviruses in malignancy. Sam Broder, the doctor who offered me a fellowship at NCI, along with another NCI investigator, Mitch Mitsuya, found a way to grow HIV (then called HTLV-3) in a test tube. Suddenly, it became possible to determine how the presence of drugs would affect the growth of AIDS.

This is a desperate time, and the institute is testing just about everything: aspirin, antibiotics, antihypertensives, various exotic compounds. Some of these drugs are then chosen for testing in patients.

Three years before I arrived, NCI had started to test drugs in a cohort of young U.S. Navy men who provide a remarkably similar description of how they contracted the disease. When their histories are taken, all claim to have been infected by a whore in the Philippines. We fellows are roughly the same age as these patients. Of course, we can surmise that the young men didn't get their HTLV-3 from a whore in the Philippines, but the fiction has to be kept up. If they admit they are gay, the young men would be given dishonorable discharges and would lose all health benefits immediately and forever.

If you are a manly man and if you get your HTLV-3 by paying for sex with a woman, the disease is deemed "service-connected." It might lead to a discharge when you get too sick to serve, but the military would take care of your medical costs for the rest of your life. However, a gay soldier or sailor would be automatically kicked out of the service.

When taking a history, the fellows would look up and, with a straight face, inquire, "The whore in the Philippines?" The young men would nod. Even those who had never set foot in the Philippines accepted this prompt.

These young men haven't received sufficient credit for their role in the wars on cancer and AIDS. Shortly before my arrival, they were among the first humans to receive AZT, the first efficacious AIDS drug. AZT was synthesized in 1964, but was shelved after being found ineffective in mice. It was revived out of desperation when NCI researchers initiated a search for something—anything—that might work against the emerging viral disease that was destroying the immune systems of homosexual men, drug addicts, and prostitutes.

In 1985, Broder starts testing AZT in humans. Largely, this means our sailors. Three years later, I would stand in the room when one of our patients—a young man from South Side Chicago—becomes the first human to receive another AIDS drug, ddI. This is a first-in-human trial, which means that the first patient receives a small dose, which, alas, turns out to be less than enough to benefit him. Both AZT and ddI are still being prescribed today.

The young men—again, primarily sailors—are also exposed to an obscure, old drug called suramin, developed in Germany in 1916 and used to treat infections caused by parasites: African sleeping sickness and river blindness. The stuff is not approved in the United States, but can be obtained through the Centers for Disease Control and Prevention.

You can see why Sam Broder would feel compelled to experiment with suramin. It's a big, glumpy molecule that looks as if it might gum up the system, blocking the AIDS virus from attaching to a receptor. In many ways, suramin is similar to AZT, an obscure compound that hardly anyone wanted. Broder tests suramin in vitro, then tries it in animals. Ultimately, the tests advance to humans.

In the setting of tropical disease, suramin causes parasites to lose energy and die. Alas, it's shown to have the same effect on humans. Young sailors succumb quickly, without discernible symptoms. They are weak and look skeletal by the time they die, and in all cases autopsies show the cause: adrenal insufficiency due to adrenal necrosis. Suramin in high doses kills off adrenal tissue.

At this point, an NCI doctor named Charles "Snuffy" Myers concludes that the adrenal connection could make suramin an important drug.

YOU could go through the NCI fellowship without seeing some common cancers. For example, in 1988, we didn't treat any colorectal cancer, the third most common cancer in the United States. I go through the program without seeing a single cancer of the pancreas, another common disease.

The cancer patients at the NIH Clinical Center are different from patients I saw at the University of Chicago and Case Western Reserve. Patients at the Clinical Center tend to be better educated and more motivated than the general population. Everyone has the diagnosis of cancer and is referred by an outside physician. This, of course, means that they have an outside physician. They are middle class or upper middle class and insured. They are folks who take an interest in their disease and an interest in their treatment. They are folks who ask questions.

However, after a few days at NCI, I realize that I am seeing a lot of adrenal-cancer patients. In the real world, adrenal cancer is exceedingly rare, a couple hundred new cases a year. You can practice oncology for forty years without seeing a single case.

Yet here they are: adrenal-cancer patients from all over the United States. I do a back-of-the-envelope calculation and realize that we are seeing half of all adrenal cancers diagnosed in the United States. We are seeing more adrenal cancer than lung cancer.

"Snuffy Myers has a Phase I protocol for suramin in adrenal cancer," a friend explains. Since autopsy studies found that several AIDS patients receiving suramin had died of adrenal necrosis, Snuffy decides that the drug that was useless in AIDS might work in adrenal cancer.

The idea seems exciting: a drug that kills patients in one setting might save lives in another. You can see how important this venture from AIDS to cancer would be for Myers, Broder, and the NCI. It would validate Broder's idea that synergies can be found in combating cancer and AIDS. This is important, because in January 1989, seven months after my arrival on campus, Broder is named to succeed DeVita as NCI director.

Snuffy, too, becomes increasingly important in the NCI hierarchy. He is named chief of a new NCI branch that combines the medicine branch and the clinical pharmacology branch. Since every fellow dreams of getting a protocol, Snuffy's aggressive thinking strikes me as a model to emulate.

Among the warlords, Snuffy's demeanor is uncharacteristically laid-back. Sandy-haired and of average height, he is approachable and pleasant. His nickname was given to him at birth. His father, also a physician, was fond of the comic-strip character Snuffy Smith, a hillbilly from southern Appalachia who detests "flatlanders" and "revenuers." When I meet him, Snuffy has a long beard, just like his comic-book alter ego.

Some doctors have CVs that sound like a symphony—deep, sustained, internally consistent. Snuffy's is more like a series of Mozart's piano sonatas. Each entry is different, each one complete. The breadth of his intellectual curiosity is astonishing, running from clinical development of the leukemia and lymphoma drug methotrexate to development of AIDS drugs. Like everyone else at NCI, he advocates the no-guts, no-glory approach to medicine: hit the thing as hard as you can, nuke it, napalm it, and damn the consequences.

His disorganization is epic. Papers in his office are arranged in piles several feet high, well beyond the point where anyone can credibly claim to know where anything is. A story is told about the time Snuffy showed up in Paris only to learn that the conference where he was scheduled to speak about suramin had ended. He gets the continent right, he gets the country right, he even gets the city right. The date, however, is wrong.

Along the way, Snuffy ends up with something no one needs: a second nickname.

"Someone named Snoopy just called you," a secretary reported to Daniel Ihde, then deputy chief of the Medical Oncology Branch at the National Naval Medical Center, an imposing New Deal tower across Rockville Pike from the NIH. Puzzled, Ihde retreats into his office to review whether he knows anyone named Snoopy. After brief pondering, Ihde reemerges from his office.

"Could it have been Snuffy?"

Snuffy, a man named after a hooting-and-hollering moonshiner, was confused with a talking, floppy-eared beagle. That was cute.

From that point on, folks at the Naval Medical Center referred to Snuffy exclusively as Snoopy.

WHEN a drug succeeds in controlling cancer, we learn about it at conferences and in scientific journals. Stories of our fiascos, though no less instructive, are almost invisible, especially if they are cautionary tales that lay bare the fundamental flaws in the system. Occasionally we'll see the data from trials where a treatment that we thought would be better actually does worse than the standard of care. Yet, in-depth analyses and narrative accounts of system failures are, almost without exception, irrevocably lost.

The story of the development of suramin has never been told in its entirety. Yet it deserves to be told, as it demonstrates the paramount importance of honesty in experimental medicine.

I was assigned to screen patients for enrollment in Snuffy's Phase I study of suramin for adrenal cancer.

Usually, before you decide on the method of administering a drug and set the dose, you determine how that drug behaves in the body. You need to know how long it lingers, how long it remains active. Typically, if a drug has a short half-life—a day—you might want to consider infusing it gradually with a pump, to keep the levels constant. If the half-life is long—say, a month—you might hit the patient with a big dose, then maintain him at a predetermined level with small doses.

When the adrenal-cancer trial started, we had no clue about suramin's pharmacokinetics, and I am not proud to admit that this gap in knowledge didn't bother me. Like Snuffy, I had bought into the war mentality. Military intel is imperfect. Pertinent facts will be established on the battlefield. From the outset, suramin was to be given to adrenal-cancer patients by continuous infusion.

As we pump suramin into adrenal-cancer patients, on day five or so some report a numbness or tingly sensation in the lips. The comments come almost as an afterthought: "Doctor, my lips feel funny."

In mid-July 1988 I hear this report—the word *complaint* is too strong—about tingly lips from a young woman named Leslie Quinn. She reports this symptom almost apologetically. She has a terminal illness, but she is determined enough and well enough connected to get on the protocol of a drug that she hopes will be the cure. I don't focus on her symptom and don't write it down.

Leslie is in her late thirties and has spectacular long, curly, dark brown hair. Her doting husband is always at her bedside. Her two lovely daughters, a teenager and a preteen, are there as well. I realize that Leslie doesn't think it's in her interest to tell us about the side effects. She is more invested in suramin than Snuffy. For Snuffy, suramin's success would be a medical breakthrough, a publication, a claim to glory. For Leslie, it's life itself.

Surely that feeling in the lips is nothing to worry about. A funny feeling is not a dose-limiting toxicity, not by itself, not usually. I am not trying to duck responsibility for the case. I had been around the block at Case Western during my residency. My clinical judgment during my time at NCI is the sharpest it would be in my entire career.

We keep the suramin pump on.

On the next morning's rounds, Leslie reports that she is unable to move her feet. She says she first had a tingling sensation in her toes, then the toes refused to take her commands. The feet are next. This is serious—peripheral neuropathy. We do the only thing we can—cut the suramin and pray. Surely, the drug is causing this reaction. Maybe without the drug the reaction will go away.

Paralysis progresses rapidly. By the next morning, thirty-six hours after things started to go awry, Leslie is in total body paralysis, hooked up to a ventilator.

The paralysis is either Guillain-Barré syndrome, an autoimmune disorder affecting the peripheral nervous system, or something similar to it. Clearly the paralysis is caused by suramin.

How did we get there? Our thinking about suramin wasn't appreciably different from our thinking about other cancer drugs. We surmised that if a small dose of an agent has a little activity, a great amount of the agent would have a lot of activity. Did we get the dose right? Is dose intensity the name of the game? Is more *really* better?

A grunt in a firefight can't stop to ponder the overarching military doctrine and geopolitical formations that catapult him across the seas. But doubts, big, dark, and fundamental, creep in after the firefight, when I am able to think. Right now I focus on keeping Leslie alive.

Our intensive care unit has no doctors. If you take a patient there, it's up to you to take care of her. I take a bed in the unit and move in with my patient. Leslie spends a week on a ventilator. When she is weaned from the ventilator, she develops pneumonia, which requires a return to the blower.

Throughout this time, Leslie's husband and I talk about immediate threats to her life. We discuss her lung function, her oxygenation, her liver, her kidneys. There is no way to predict whether she will pull through. We take fire. We incur casualties. Some are wounded, some are killed.

Leslie is paralyzed for about two weeks. She requires physical and occupational therapy to learn to move her arms and legs again. She never regains the ability to walk independently.

Researching this book, I learned that at the time I was treating Leslie, our colleagues at the Naval hospital were horrified to hear stories about our suramin adrenal-cancer trial. They knew that patients were ending up in the ICU with the Guillain-Barré syndrome, and that we didn't—weren't willing to—stop the trial and see whether we could at least get the toxicity under control.

Snuffy's nickname Snoopy was taking deeper roots across Rockville Pike. The image of the dog wandering onto dangerous terrain and unexpectedly encountering the fearsome Guillain-Barré syndrome (or a condition that mimics it) made observers smirk through puzzlement and sadness.

Looking back, I don't know why we didn't stop the trial, even temporarily. We had good reasons to be humble. At the time, we had no assay for measuring the levels of suramin in the blood and no way to know how long the drug stayed in the body. Maybe we were afraid of the answers. Maybe we thought we already had the answers. Instead of acknowledging the limits of our knowledge, we forged ahead, blindly pushing toward what we hoped was the cure.

Leslie's symptoms and illness didn't cause us to rethink the wisdom of continuing the trial. Eventually, experiences such as hers helped us figure out that half the patients making the lips-feel-funny complaint didn't progress to paralysis if the drug was stopped. Also, experiences of patients such as Leslie helped us learn to measure the level of suramin in the blood and pinpoint the level at which the drug caused Guillain-Barré syndrome.

My work with Snuffy and the suramin trial ends in 1989. I rotate to the Naval Medical Center and then to two years of research when I start to focus on issues of public health and cancer prevention.

I do learn a lesson from Snuffy. He confirms the truth I learned as a kid: doctors try out things just to see whether they will work. Here is the Great Snuffy Myers—chief of the Clinical Pharmacology Branch of the premier cancer-research institution in the world—doing what poor, illiterate factory workers in Detroit were telling me to look out for when I was nine years old.

Chapter 14

How Much Protection?

THE POWER OF CANCER to kill is so fearsome that treating it naturally invites the metaphor of war. As oncologists, we crave big weapons and are eager to throw them into the field. This is our mind-set, our history, our culture. Sometimes it's also our folly, our madness.

Some of the key strategies that still guide us can be traced to the NCI of the 1950s and 1960s, when two young doctors with strikingly similar names—Emil "J" Freireich and Emil "Tom" Frei—performed a series of experiments on children dying of acute leukemia.

The leukemia ward at NCI at the time was terrifying. The blood on the sheets was the first thing one noticed—children were routinely bleeding to death. Mortality from the disease was 100 percent.

In 1955, Freireich came up with an idea for controlling the hemorrhages: give the kids platelets. Shockingly to people who thought they understood blood, Freireich was determined to skip a step. He didn't want to waste time on testing his theories in animals. He would go directly to the kids.

First, J tried thawed-out, previously frozen platelets. When he gave this treatment to a child, the bleeding stopped, albeit for five minutes or so. So, J decided to try fresh platelets.

Hematologists told him it was completely insane. J's opponents made the—seemingly logical—case that if you infuse fresh platelets even once, the patient would become sensitized, which would render the intervention impossible in the future.

J transfused platelets without formal consent, without protocols, without approval of any board responsible for monitoring ethics and safety; indeed, he did it without any formal safeguards. This was 1955. The concept of "informed consent" did not fully enter medicine until years later. At that time, doctors still knew best, and no forms were required. (Even drugs were still being approved based on their "purity." Proof of effectiveness was not needed.) If you owned a white coat, you could pursue your hunches.

No one knows how well these children and their parents understood the experiments and the risks. Did the scientists conducting the experiments tell the kids or their parents that they had no earthly idea what was about to happen? Did Freireich and Frei even understand that they had no rational way to predict the outcome? It seems that at best the doctors explained how excited they were about their hypothesis, and permission would follow. What else was there to do? These were desperate parents of dying children.

Fortunately, this time skeptics in the hematology establishment were wrong and J's approach worked. When leukemia patients were given fresh platelets, their bleeding stopped.

After finding a way to stop the bleeding, Freireich and Frei came up with another wild idea: combine all the drugs that were at the time used to treat the disease. They used four drugs: vincristine, amethopterin, mercaptopurine, and prednisone, abbreviated as VAMP. This regimen was a witch's brew, a combination of nasty drugs, each with a different mechanism of action and different side effects. They wanted to administer it at a maximum strength, and they wanted to continue to treat their patients after the point where visible signs of disease had disappeared.

The approach of hitting the disease with multiple drugs, each with a different way of attacking the cancer, became known as combination chemotherapy. It's logical, sort of: if you can give multiple active drugs that attack the cancer cell at several different points of vulnerability, you get more activity than with one drug. More activity in this case means more cancer cells dying. Following this naturally is the idea of administering drugs at the maximum tolerated dose. Administering large doses of chemotherapy drugs became known as dose-intensive chemotherapy.

These approaches—flying by the seat of your pants, combining everything under the sun, and continuing to treat even after the signs of the disease are gone—continued to guide Snuffy et al. a quarter of a century after Freireich and Frei, when I arrived at NCI.

Fast-forward another quarter century, and we still use combination therapies, often administering new, expensive, targeted drugs with the old warhorses of oncology, drugs that have now been around longer than some of the oncologists prescribing them.

We still conduct early-phase research to determine the side effects to set the "maximum tolerated dose" of just about every new drug. We still argue about optimal strategies for stopping treatment: how long do we continue to treat after all visible signs of disease disappear?

Do we continue to treat after therapy appears to have failed?

MANY observers predicted that VAMP would be horrendously toxic and would end in disaster, which indeed seemed to occur when several of the kids treated at NCI ended up in comas and on ventilators.

Yet, the kids recovered, and biopsies of the bone marrow showed that they were free of disease. Could VAMP have been the cure for childhood leukemia?

There was much rejoicing, which came to a halt after several kids started to develop new neurological problems. These problems led doctors to discover that in most cases VAMP wasn't curing leukemia. Instead, some of the disease was hiding behind the protection of the blood-brain barrier. These kids relapsed with disease in their brains. About 5 percent of the children survived for more than a year, and only a small number of treated children, for reasons no one understands, became long-term survivors.

THROUGHOUT his long career, Freireich has sided with organizations that argue that a dying patient should not be impeded from taking any risk he or she chooses. Predominantly, these are political conservatives who object to the requirement by FDA that clinical researchers obtain "investigational new drug" licenses before administering an experimental therapy. An IND is given after the drug sponsor has presented data to the FDA demonstrating that the drug can be tested safely. The FDA does not require any proof of efficacy to grant an IND. Clinical trials done under an IND ultimately develop the data, which the drug's developer eventually takes to the FDA to get a new drug approved. Incredibly, the editorial board of *The Wall Street Journal* has spent the past five decades railing against the FDA requirement that pharmaceutical companies demonstrate that their products are effective in fighting disease.

To conservatives, these requirements, enacted in 1962, are the juncture in history when things went terribly wrong, a kind of a regulatory equivalent of the original sin. The same groups also mount ethical challenges to placebo-controlled randomized trials, arguing that it's morally wrong to withhold a treatment from half of your patients.

Freireich has often said that the nanny state personified by the FDA bureaucrats has no business inserting itself into the doctor-patient relationship. As an octogenarian physician at MD Anderson Cancer Center in Houston, J continues to argue against big government getting involved in the clinic. A few years ago, J joined a group called the Abigail Alliance for Better Access to Experimental Drugs, which sought to make drugs available immediately after they pass through Phase I testing.

Phase I studies establish the maximally tolerated dose and side effects. The primary aim of a Phase I trial is not to determine whether the drug benefits the patient. Indeed, only 5 percent of cancer drugs show anticancer activity in Phase I testing. Effectiveness is determined in Phase II studies.

The group's campaign resulted in a court case that was upheld by a three-judge panel at the U.S. Court of Appeals for the District of Columbia. Ultimately, a panel of all judges seated on that court rejected that petition, and the Supreme Court refused to reconsider the appellate court's ruling.

In the heat of that battle, Freireich spoke to a reporter about his frustration with the power of the FDA. "They can't regulate the interaction between a physician-scientist and a dying cancer patient," he said to *The Cancer Letter* in 2005. "That is something that is in the area of professional expertise, and they don't know shit about it. You give power to an agency, the agency has to find people who will do this drone work, so they look for failed oncologists, and the failed oncologists love this position, because now they have power."

FDA is just one component of regulatory oversight of clinical trials. In an interview with *The Cancer Letter,* Freireich was particularly angry about the role of his former MD Anderson colleague Richard Pazdur, a colorectal-cancer expert who left for Washington to become head of the FDA's cancer unit. Pazdur is a favorite target of attacks by the Abigail Alliance and *The Wall Street Journal* editors.

"Look at Ricky Pazdur!" Freireich continued. "He was so-so and not doing much; now he is King Kong! He gets invited to every talk on every drug at every meeting everywhere in the world. Who would know what is the highest probability of benefiting a patient and the lowest probability of doing harm? Is it Dr. Pazdur, who's been sitting at a desk for ten years, or is it Dr. Freireich, who's in the clinic, beating his ass, taking care of dying cancer patients? Who knows more about this?

"What is wrong with us? The system is upside down!"

I find it interesting that Freireich's political position is rooted in his early success, which indisputably paved the way toward the cure of childhood leukemia. Had success stories driven by instinct been the norm rather than an exception, Freireich's argument would have supported elimination of any and all efforts to ensure that patients are told the truth and are protected from exploitation, whether it's motivated by financial greed on the part of a private doctor or eagerness on the part of an academic to find another subject for a clinical trial.

Alas, such triumphs are not often repeated. Instead, the scenario most frequently replicated in drug development is better illustrated by suramin.

I got to know J in the early 1990s, when he spent a year on sabbatical at the NCI. Tall, heavy, solid, and in his seventies, he was approachable and friendly. He joked that MD Anderson had sent him into exile (this was true), and NCI director Sam Broder had asked him to study the training of medical oncologists.

J's sense of humor takes a while to get used to. Once, in front of me, he said to my mentor Peter Greenwald, then director of the NCI Division of Cancer Prevention and Control, "We finally find a good one and you pervert him by convincing him to be interested in this prevention shit."

The word *one* in "a good one" stood for "Negro." This backhanded compliment threw me back on my heels for a moment, as I had rarely experienced racism from doctors.

The second half of J's joke was equally shocking: the gullible mind of this just-discovered "good one"—Otis—was being corrupted with dangerous teachings about cancer prevention and all the nonsense that goes into it.

For starters, J dismissed the concept of public health. He went on to expound on his contempt for Phase III trials. These trials compare two treatments to determine which is better. "When a treatment works, it is obvious that it works, and you don't need a study to show it," he said. Then he went on to slam prevention, a discipline highly dependent on Phase III trials, many of them involving placebo.

Finally, on the off chance that he was being too subtle, J explained that public health is self-evidently an absurd concept. "When a group of people is stranded on a desert island, they decide which of them is going to *treat* disease. They don't decide who is going to *prevent* disease."

As the conversation progressed, I let go of my initial feeling of outrage. I understood that this was J being J. Our conversation demonstrated another manifestation of his unusual sense of humor and a bit of the outrageousness that has punctuated his career. Yet, two decades later, Greenwald still remembers being shaken by this conversation.

I am still fond of J and have considered him a friend for more than twenty years. He is an icon of oncology. I may even share some of his penchant for in-your-face truth-telling. Throwing hardballs in the debates of medicine is a fair tactic. (All is fair in efforts to provoke people to think.) However, I disagree with J's contention that the research world is upside down.

I don't know how you can responsibly practice medicine without measuring effectiveness of therapies you are administering. We have to know that the treatments we are testing are better than standard treatments or nothing at all. Without the requirement that drugs demonstrate effectiveness, we simply cannot know whether we are doing harm.

In the case of drugs for diseases where we have treatments but no cure, only randomization will give you the answer.

I share J's frustration that many of our successes increase median survival by three or four months at best. I have never talked to J about it, but I was thinking of him when the combination of Gemzar and Tarceva was approved by the FDA for cancer of the pancreas, because in a clinical trial it increased median survival by fourteen days.

Our progress is not fast enough.

RESPONSIBLE medical researchers recognize that by definition we are dealing with the unknown. We put patients at risk while we hope to do good. Often—particularly in Phase I studies—we struggle with a profound dilemma: Whom are we trying to benefit? Are we trying to benefit the patient in front of us? Or are we trying to benefit society, which may benefit from knowledge gained through the experiment we are conducting? We try to be decent and respectful, and here Father Polakowski's maxim fits particularly well. We try to explain the truth about the experiment: what are the known risks, what is not known, and what is believed.

For a Phase I trial, you have to know enough to believe that the experiment has merit. You can't cut corners—you have to find out everything you possibly can before you put a patient in harm's way. If you are testing a drug, for example, you can't rush into a study without learning as much about the drug as you can in preclinical studies.

When doing a human study, you also have to have what ethicists call equipoise. It is unethical to put a patient on a study if you are convinced you know the answer. If you are convinced that Drug A is better than Drug B, it is unethical to give a patient Drug B.

Ultimately, this ability to say truthfully, genuinely, and sincerely that you don't know is the principal distinction between responsible research and the wilderness.

The very nature of what we do requires a good clinical researcher to have a certain amount of ego, perhaps even a touch of hubris. If you are a patient, you do not want an insecure, uncertain physician. This is even more important when you are in a clinical study. As a practical matter, it's important to have objective third parties look over the investigator's shoulder, to make sure that he hasn't fallen in love with his own ideas, that he isn't cutting corners.

It's okay to have beliefs—you need them to formulate the scientific question, the hypothesis, you are testing—but they have to be labeled as such. It's also important to make sure that someone knowledgeable and objective is overseeing the researcher and that this person—or this committee—is willing to ask tough questions.

As cancer doctors, we are in no position to promise the cure. But we do have the moral obligation to tell the truth. My stake in a clinical study is different from my patients'. I stand to gain publication in a medical journal, meet my financial quota for selling clinical services (most institutions have those), maintain my cancer center, receive a federal grant, or perhaps earn consulting fees from a drug company. A patient could end up experiencing longer survival or a catastrophic toxicity. If I want to be able to look at myself in the mirror, I have to be certain that my patients have a clear understanding of my scientific justification for conducting the clinical experiment as well as my understanding of its potential risks and benefits.

I have to be certain that I have done all I can to explain uncertainty to my patients. Any shortcut in that endeavor amounts to denying my patients' humanity and my own.

Chapter 15

The Guillain-Barré Syndrome

BEFORE SCREENING PATIENTS for the suramin study, I glance at the protocol and see that it's a classic Phase I, which means that we would begin by treating three patients at a dose we believe to be too low. Then, if they do well, we would double the dose and treat another cohort of three patients. And so forth until we slam into a dose-limiting toxicity. In the beginning, you hurt people by not giving them enough drug. In the end, you hurt people by giving too much. When you get to that point, you scale back the dose to the maximum beneficial amount.

As we screen patients, we verify the staging of their adrenal cancer, review pathology, and generally make sure they do indeed have adrenal cancer. Those whose disease is metastatic to the liver or lung are put on suramin.

During screening I notice for the first time that patients at NCI are remarkably optimistic about their chances of getting a cure. This is puzzling in a Phase I trial, where the goal is to find the right dose for later studies. Benefiting the patients, let alone *curing* them, is not the goal at this stage; sure, it could happen by accident, but we aren't tailoring the experiment to this end. The question we are asking is limited: how much of this glumpy substance can we give to a human before triggering a catastrophic event?

The question of benefit would have to wait till the next phases—Phase II and Phase III—of development. Health benefits—if any—would be more likely to accrue later, most likely not to patients getting the drug in Phase I.

After putting Leslie on a ventilator, I start to wonder whether we—the researchers—are failing to tell these patients the truth. Are we delineating what we know from what we don't know and from what we believe? Or are these patients not paying attention, deliberately refusing to hear? Whatever the explanation, do these patients understand the risks they are taking? Do they understand the likelihood of benefits? Are they lying to themselves or are they being duped?

In 1995, researchers at the University of Chicago published a study that demonstrates just how poorly patients understand the risks and benefits of Phase I studies. A team led by oncologist and bioethicist Christopher Daugherty surveyed thirty patients who enrolled in a Phase I trial. Their finding was astonishing: 85 percent of patients chose the trial in pursuit of therapeutic benefit. Worse, only a third of the patients were able to restate the purpose of the trial in which they were enrolled. Together, these findings suggest that a minority of patients in such studies have a clear understanding of the risks they have agreed to take.

Exceedingly rarely does a physician pull a patient off a Phase I protocol for ethical reasons. I would see it happen only once—at NCI, when an AIDS patient who had tried three courses of therapy became obsessed with the fourth. His enthusiasm was sparked by something called a molecular sponge, or CD-4. The idea was to fool the AIDS virus to bind to an intravenously administered receptor rather than the patient's cells. The Phase I protocol in this case served to uncover the maximum amount of the molecular sponge a patient could tolerate.

The patient badly wanted to receive the sponge, and he clearly not only hoped that he would get better but seemed to be *expecting* that he would get better. He talked so much to fellows and the nurses that we went to the principal investigator on the trial and informed him of an ethical problem with putting that patient on the trial.

We cringed at the thought of contradicting the patient's desires, but ultimately we were looking after his welfare. This was someone who expected more than could be promised, someone who didn't comprehend the gamble he was about to take. Once on therapy, he could become so invested that he would not report side effects, potentially sustaining harm. And in the end, he would almost certainly have to face the disappointment of drug failure.

Although J Freireich would have had no problem with this state of affairs, some of my NCI colleagues and I did. The principal investigator on the trial—Robert Yarchoan, Broder's collaborator on AIDS work—took our concerns seriously and went to see the patient. Yarchoan tried to explain the goals and limitations of the therapy. They spoke several times, but Yarchoan's message didn't seem to get through. Finally, he decided that it would be unethical to offer the patient the molecular sponge. This decision taught us, the fellows, an important lesson about ethics in research: it's wrong to be anxious to put patients on trials. Safeguards matter.

Of course, the patient was gravely disappointed. But he was not deprived of the cure. The therapy was ultimately shown to be ineffective.

THE study of suramin in adrenal cancer went nowhere, too, but Snuffy thought of another use for the agent—prostate cancer. With time, Snuffy and his team learned to measure the levels of the drug in the blood. As a result, they learned that the Guillain-Barré syndrome sets in when the drug level reaches 300 mcg/ml of blood serum.

To manage toxicity, Snuffy proposed rigorous monitoring. He called it "adaptive control with feedback." It was so complicated that only NCI would dare to attempt it. Clinical pharmacologists outside NCI called the approach mumbo jumbo. They saw it as just another case of NCI hubris, insistence that the institute's scientists know what they are doing even if it makes no sense to anyone else in the field.

The drug seemed to have another toxicity. It was a blood thinner, a lot like Coumadin. Patients had to be counseled to avoid shaving or banging their fists against tables—any activity that might ordinarily result in cuts and bruises.

Snuffy also learned that suramin has an unusually long half-life—fifty days. This means that it takes fifty days for half of the drug to be excreted from the patient's body. Usually, a drug with a long half-life is administered quickly with an "induction dose," then kept up at the therapeutic level with small doses. Yet, for reasons that surprised many of his colleagues in clinical pharmacology, Snuffy decided to keep the slow infusion regimen intact. The objective was to get as close as possible to 300 mcg/ml because more is, of course, better.

Snuffy's hypothesis was based on an observation of drops in PSA levels in some metastatic prostate cancer patients whose disease returns despite treatment with hormones. Snuffy took them off hormones—at that time, flutamide—and gave them suramin and the steroid prednisone. (The prednisone was added to replace the steroids that their bodies were unable to produce because the patients' adrenal glands had, literally, died.) Indeed, after a while, some of these patients experienced drops in their PSA levels.

If you looked only at how you gave the patient suramin and his PSA went down, you might conclude that you had the cure. Unless, of course, nature was giving us the middle finger and we were unable to recognize it.

Chapter 16

Saving Representative Silvio Conte

AN ARGUMENT can be made that no one on Capitol Hill will ever believe in the War on Cancer more passionately than Congressman Silvio O. Conte, a liberal Republican representing a largely Democratic district in the Berkshire hills of western Massachusetts. As a ranking member of the House Appropriations Committee, Conte is among the most valuable friends NCI can ask for.

Conte is an American original. He is a son of Italian immigrants. He is a World War II veteran. He is an avid hunter and fisherman. He loves cigars. He has grandchildren who call him Nonno. He grows tomatoes in the backyard of his Bethesda home. He gives away the crops. He drives a hot-red Pontiac GTO. He is fiercely independent. Though a Republican, he voted against the resolution that enabled President George H. W. Bush to enter the first Persian Gulf War.

In 1987, Conte is diagnosed with prostate cancer. The disease is found early enough for surgeons at Johns Hopkins University to remove his prostate. In 1988, he gets additional surgery, to replace a knee ruined as a result of a football injury. That surgery lands him in an electric cart, which he promptly decorates with Italian and American flags. He is especially fond of the cart's horn, which he blasts with abandon in the hallways of the Capitol.

The cancer progresses rapidly. It becomes obvious that his tumor was not localized, as the surgeon had hoped. Conte goes on a hormonal treatment. This works for a while. However, in December 1990, Conte is told that the treatment has failed him. A doctor at Hopkins advises the sixty-nine-year-old congressman to get his affairs in order.

Conte's daughter Michelle recalls her father calling her in tears. "I just can't believe this, I can't believe this," he keeps repeating. Michelle calls the doctor at Hopkins, who repeats to her that Conte should get his house in order, and that Michelle and other family members should be guiding him in that direction.

Conte doesn't want to give up. First, he goes to see Fernand Labrie, a Canadian endocrinologist. The journey in a small plane proves difficult. After going to see Labrie, Conte calls Michelle and says, "I am so tired, it was brutal."

The Canadian doctor sees no hope in the situation. "I wish we had never gone," Conte's wife, Corinne, says to Michelle.

At the time, NCI's Phase I/II trial of suramin is hard to miss as the final shot at hormone-refractory prostate cancer. NCI officials trumpet the drug's promise far and wide, and for a man in Conte's position—that of an appropriator—the trumpeting would be deafening.

I don't know whether that was the case with Conte, but I do know that NCI officials make special efforts to recruit sick politicians. Conte has sharp political instincts. Educated to think critically by Jesuits at Boston College, he has no fear of questioning accepted truths. He is able to foresee the military quagmire of Vietnam. He has the courage to vote his conscience on Iraq.

Why doesn't he say no to suramin? Does his belief in the conquest of cancer and his personal contact with the generals leading that war dull his otherwise sensitive bullshit gauge?

"He was a sitting duck for that," daughter Michelle says. "He firmly believed in the NCI mission. We've got the best, we are cutting-edge. He was always into the newest thing. He had all these friends. He was always approached as someone who could provide. That was his position. He was in appropriations."

Conte has access to top-notch experts in defense, but no access to state-of-the-art clinical pharmacologists.

As a fellow at NCI, I, too, was a believer in the promise of suramin, or at least enough of an agnostic that I could be involved in testing it in patients. I was not directly involved in Conte's care. I think his story is illustrative of a problem in medicine, and it is told with permission of his daughter.

It's not clear how much the Conte family knows about the risks and benefits of suramin. "My mother was a nurse," Michelle says in an interview nearly two decades later. "She didn't know the risks." Corinne Conte would have understood the risks, and in the close-knit Conte family, she would have told the kids.

On February 1, 1991, Conte starts to experience paralysis, and Corinne calls a military appropriations aide and an administrative assistant to help her take him to NIH.

"He was having a horrible headache and feeling weak, very weak," Michelle says.

A CT scan reveals a blood clot near the right side of Conte's brain. Without doubt, this was caused by suramin, which thins the blood and increases the risk of bleeding. Surgery is planned.

The day before surgery, Conte's mind runs along two tracks. There is the cheerful, positive persona. "He was talking about going to Florida after NIH," says Michelle. "He thought he would make it through, and he had been working on the National Archives project in Pittsfield." The archives would contain his papers. He brings a briefcase to NIH, and he works a little.

He also has an intense conversation with Corinne. This larger-than-life American accepts that death is near. "He had a premonition before going into that surgery about coming out," Michelle says. "He said to her before he went in, 'Corinne, don't hook me up to anything. I want to go. I don't want to be hooked up to machines.'"

NIH surgeons attempt to remove the clot, but the operation fails. Another blood clot develops almost immediately, putting Conte into a coma.

"He was never conscious," Michelle recalls. "They had him completely bandaged up, and there was some bleeding coming through it. He kept twitching, his arms kept moving up and down, but I know he could hear us."

As the appropriator's life slips away, NCI doctors push for another surgery. "NIH people were saying, 'We can do it, we can keep him going. He will come back. We can see him driving his GTO down the road, waving.' They were talking about keeping him on life support," Michelle recalls. A local urologist, a personal friend, joins the family to provide perspective, support, and sober guidance.

Michelle remembers being horrified. These people wanted to fight, fight, fight, denying defeat. "This was bizarre," Michelle recalls. "What in the heck is wrong with these people?"

Finally the urologist friend speaks up. "If this were my father, I would let him go now. There is no real hope of him ever having a normal life. Half of his brain is damaged. He will never be able to be Silvio again."

The family, too, decides to honor Silvio's wishes and not go through with another surgery. The congressman dies in his hospital bed a week after being wheeled into the Clinical Center.

IT took more than a decade, but science did a fine job of sorting though Snuffy's beliefs about suramin, demonstrating that they are, without exception, wrong. First, Snuffy's observation that suramin decreases the PSA level in hormone-refractory prostate cancer—Conte's disease—was incorrect. Howard Scher, of Memorial Sloan-Kettering Cancer Center, published a paper in the *Journal of Clinical Oncology* in 1993 that struck at the heart of Snuffy's reasoning. Scher's research reported that merely withdrawing hormone-refractory patients from flutamide, a hormonal therapy, decreased their PSA levels.

Here is how it works: At first, the tumor hates flutamide, but over time, it learns to like it, even grow from it. Stop flutamide, and the disease will slow down for a while. This was not the cure. It was flutamide withdrawal. Snuffy stumbled upon it and Scher described it.

The change in PSA—which Snuffy believed to be an indicator of clinical improvement—isn't worth much. It's a measurement made in a lab. It doesn't necessarily mean anything to an actual patient. Your PSA could go down, and you may not know the difference. The FDA has never accepted a drop in PSA as a criterion for approving prostate-cancer drugs.

Another study compared three doses of suramin and showed conclusively that there is no relationship between intensity of the dose and the drug's effect. The study, by Eric Small et al., published in the *Journal of*

Clinical Oncology in 2002, showed that suramin at any dose—high, intermediate, or low—produced the same impact on survival and progression of disease. However, toxicity was more severe at high doses. More was worse.

I don't understand how any pharmaceutical company could believe that suramin could make a plausible drug. Yet Parke-Davis did. It took extraordinary courage as well as a deep denial of reality for the company to file an application for suramin after a clinical trial had shown that patients on placebo were living longer than patients receiving suramin. On October 1, 1998, the FDA's advisers voted 10–0 against approval of the Parke-Davis application, and the agency accepted their recommendation.

Meanwhile, NIH honored Conte's memory. A building housing child health and neuroscience research now bears his name.

"Isn't it ironic?" says his daughter Michelle. "He died of complications to the brain and they name a brain-research building after him."

Chapter 17

The Quintessential American

I AM AT THE ATLANTA AIRPORT, picking up phone messages that piled up while I was in the air. The volume of calls is insane, and not all of them are interesting.

I get a lot of internal ACS policy inquiries. What should we say about an issue that's about to come up in Congress? Do we jump in now, do we wait a bit, or do we stay out? A lot of calls deal with ethics issues. Should employee X be allowed to do outside consulting? What if it's without pay?

I get calls from Capitol Hill aides, off-the-record, because the senator wants to understand the issues before mouthing off. Then there are calls from reporters; a few of them have my cell phone number. Sometimes it's about a story. Other times it's about Grandpa in Tennessee. He has prostate cancer and needs to see someone good.

My rule in triaging calls is to put patient-related matters first. (In this hypothetical lineup, the reporter with the sick grandfather in Tennessee gets my callback first.)

And when a message starts "Dr. Brawley, Alan Rabson suggested that I call . . . ," this is all I need to triage this call to the top, even above the old guy in Tennessee. This is my opportunity to practice medicine in its pure form, to save someone from the jaws of the system, to stop a medical travesty, maybe even save a life.

On an average day, my work has internal logic, intrinsic flow. There is legislation to track, reporters to set on the path of seeing the world as it is, advocates who need to be reminded that the rules of evidence don't change. Alas, this flow of activity makes it easy to forget that my business is about helping people.

One of the greatest honors a human can bestow upon another is to say, "Can you help me?" When you do help someone, you get an incredible feeling of satisfaction. When you make a big difference, you get a high. Al Rabson helps me experience this satisfaction.

Al is a superb pathologist, a retired admiral in the Public Health Service, a veteran of more than half a century of combat against cancer. Even now, in his eighties, he retains the title of deputy director of the National Cancer Institute.

I worry about Al. His wife, the NIH scientist and administrator Ruth Kirschstein, died of multiple myeloma recently. They were a power couple. They lived for their work, but with every subtle movement showed how much they cared about each other. I worry about how long Al will last without Ruth's calm, determined presence.

Aging has not been kind to PHS's Rear Admiral Upper Half (ret.) Alan Rabson. He needs a walker to get around and is mostly confined to the redbrick, two-bedroom, government-owned house behind the tall fence of the NIH campus. In his decline, Al hasn't been relying on friends. Few have been ushered in to see him. Mostly it's "the practice" that keeps Al going.

The practice began in 1955, when he came to NCI following a pathology fellowship at Tulane University. The way Al tells it, shortly after he moved into his office, the phone rang. The call was from a woman he didn't know. He isn't even sure how she got his name, but he does remember her question: "I have breast cancer. Whom shall I go to see?"

"I sent her to a doctor I knew, who did a lot of breast cancer," Al recalled recently. "And because I was at the Cancer Institute, I knew a lot of people. And I read widely, so I knew who was doing what."

Word started to get out that a knowledgeable doctor at NCI was answering the patients' questions—and that you could call him as often as you needed to. The scenario is always the same: a voice on the phone stumbles through the words on the pathology report. Al hears this halting, stuttering speech, and the words have an effect that can best be portrayed in a comic novel: an imaginary light flashes, and a tumor appears in a bubble above Al's head.

"As a pathologist, I can see the tumors in my mind."

He explains the tumor, describes the course the disease will take, lists the options for interventions, the rationale, the hope. Al is always hopeful—more so than I—because hope is better than the alternative, and because he is a better man than I am.

Al doesn't care whether he is being asked to help a multimillionaire news anchor, a US senator, or an immigrant taxi driver. "They are fellow humans, and I usually don't inquire too seriously about whether they are human," Al said recently. "Usually, I find out who sent them to me, out of curiosity, not that it matters."

As he provides a referral, Al makes sure that the patient knows that the first phrase out of his mouth should be "Al Rabson suggested that I call you."

"Of course, I never refer without telling them that they can say that I sent them," Al said. His list of doctors is enormous, and he knows how each of them thinks. That's because he trained many of them. He gets feedback, too, as patients from his practice call back to check in and tell Al how their treatment is going.

"I try to find something not too far away, but also someone who is good. I won't send them to anyone unless I trust them. I give them names. I say, 'You can go talk with them, see if you are pleased with them.' But in the end, they will have to make their own decision." Sometimes, Al admits, when a patient is about to make a choice he disagrees with, he nudges along with pointed questions, Socratically.

A referral from Al gets you an appointment immediately—and you get a callback from the doctor rather than a nurse or a clerk at the appointment desk. This is in part because the doctors on his list see his practice as a kind of guaranteed safe passage for the lucky few who stumble upon Al, and in part because all of us want to remain on his list of good docs.

A patient can call Al again and again, as often as necessary. It's illegal for Al to charge for his guidance, not that he would want to. Asking whether there is any way to return the favor earns a chuckle of the sort only an impish Jewish man can produce. I think it means Al wants you to return the favor by living a long life and being kind to others, but this is left unsaid.

No one knows how many people have benefited from Al's guidance. He gets at least one call per day, sometimes three or more. Nothing is logged, and no notes are kept. Assuming one call per patient per day, including weekends (a fair assumption), over fifty-five years, you get 20,075 patients. The actual number is certainly much larger.

In a conversation recently Al said that he worries about succession. His practice is about personal contacts, and about the quality of specialists on his list. He knows who is good, he knows whom to avoid. "I've been at the cancer institute for fiftysomething years, getting to know all these people, many of whom have gone on to fame and glory," he says. "Who else would have training like that? I can't give that to anybody."

I return the call.

It's from a scientist at NIH. His sister, who is in her midforties and lives in Atlanta, has early-stage colon cancer. He says simply, "My sister is seeing some doctors, and she needs help in assimilating what she should be doing. Would you talk to her?" In retrospect, I realize that trepidation was in his voice, but this is not at all clear in the moment.

"Would she be interested in talking to me?" I ask, because sometimes people want you to intervene in cases where intervention is inappropriate. The patient has to want to initiate contact and want to hear what you have to say.

"Can I give you her phone number?"

"I don't want her phone number," I say. "You give her my cell phone number, tell her to call me, and it's best to call me after six p.m., because that way we can sit down and spend some time talking."

I am under the impression that she needs to make some decisions, that she has some questions. Cancer is hard to understand, and doctors rush patients. Most of the time, helping Al Rabson's patients means slowing them down long enough so they can understand the treatment choices.

I get a call at 7:00 p.m. the next evening. I am at home, helping my daughters, Laura and Alison, with their homework. My kids have gotten used to seeing Daddy giving them time and then, all of a sudden, getting called away to do something patient-related. When this happens, I go to my basement office so they don't hear any of the details. This protects the kids and the patients' confidentiality.

My basement office is my favorite place in the house. My two computers are there, sitting on two computer desks. One of the computers has two big screens; it's there to let me write, check my e-mail, and listen to a Washington news-radio station I like. (I haven't switched my news junkie's loyalty to Atlanta stations.) My second computer gets used exclusively for doing lit searches when I write.

The scanner and three printers—the color printer, the photo printer, and the laser printer—are in the basement office, too. I am a techno fiend, so everything is networked. There is also a fully extended, Danish, teak dining-room table, which I bought at a Washington furniture store called Scan some thirty years ago. (I was single at the time; Yolanda favors more traditional designs.) The table is covered with objects that rule my everyday life.

The heavy-duty stapler is there, prominent, indispensable. More important than the stapler is my eight-inch-thick pile of classic papers on cancer screening. I refer to them regularly, and they are dog-eared to various extents. They are not in any order, but I know how to find what I need. There is also a pile of papers I intend to read if I ever get the time, and a pile of receipts I need for preparing income taxes.

Since the surface of the table is full, journals and books end up on the floor. They are in neat piles, but they are on the floor. The kids don't come in because they don't want to knock over the piles. The place is not a mess, just full. I clean regularly.

My favorite artwork is here, too: the crocheted portrait of me that Helen Williams made when I was treating her, and a poster of Robert F. Kennedy sailing a small boat off Cape Cod. I love the image and the RFK motto beneath it: "One man can make a difference, and every man should try."

With my cell phone in my ear, I settle into a comfortable desk chair and listen to the young woman on the other end. Her name is Debbie Kurtz. As she speaks, my mind constructs the image of her as a together forty-seven-year-old woman with a big mane of curly hair. She lives in Sandy Springs, a new-money Atlanta suburb. I imagine her in a silver Range Rover, driving kids to soccer games.

We go through the usual dance steps. She is polite, but it's clear that the honorific doesn't intimidate her; she is comfortable with access. "Dr. Brawley, thank you for talking to me," and so forth. I do my usual, telling her not to call me Dr., I go by Otis.

I ask her what's going on, and she tells me that she was diagnosed with Dukes' A colon cancer. I breathe a sigh of relief. Dukes' A is early disease. Chances are, this woman will be around for years to come.

She tells me that she is looking at all options to make sure that the cancer doesn't come back. She tells me who operated on her. I know the guy; she is in an excellent referral network. The surgeon, John Mason, is not an academic, but he is fine. An interesting inequity exists in medicine. Academic doctors generally don't refer patients to nonacademics, while nonacademics refer to academics all the time Some of us think that nonacademics aren't as good as us, not as up-to-date on literature. However, some great docs only see patients, and Mason is one of them.

I ask how she was diagnosed, and she tells me that she had blood in her stools and got a colonoscopy. A large polyplike mass was biopsied, and it showed adenocarcinoma.

We talk briefly about her and her background. I see that Debbie is intelligent, motivated. Early on, she lets it slip that she went to one of the Seven Sisters colleges. She is educated, active, and has used her brain and connections to get the best care. I see no reason to doubt anything she says.

She has her medical records in front of her. I ask her to read the surgery report. John Mason dictates a wonderful op report. It almost merits a place in American literature. As Debbie reads the notes, I can actually visualize the surgery. Mason talks about a vertical incision through the skin, going through the layers of the abdomen, finding the bowel, isolating the area where the tumor is, clamping off both sides, resecting out the arteries and veins. He talks about putting a barrier underneath the bowel, so the bowel contents don't spill into the abdomen. He talks about cutting the bowel and carefully removing it from the abdomen. A great surgery beautifully described.

The pathology report is beautiful, too. They dissected out a goodly number of lymph nodes: eighteen. One way I know someone had good service is by the number of nodes analyzed. If the path report says three of four lymph nodes, that means the surgeon didn't do an adequate operation or the pathologist was lazy. Debbie's tumor on the pathology was just in the first layer of the bowel, which made it a low-stage disease, no vascular invasion, no invasion of lymphatics. I am not as good as Al Rabson at visualizing tumors, but I can discern that Debbie had an excellent surgery and an excellent examination of pathology.

The medical oncologist on the case is Dina Habib, a young doctor born in Egypt, but educated in US medical schools. By the patient's story, Habib was thorough and nice. I agree with Dina Habib's recommendation for follow-up: a colonoscopy in one year and a CT in six months and then annually, with blood studies every six months. She suggests that the patient might want to talk to a genetic counselor, although with the lack of family history, genetic testing would not be recommended.

Habib noted that Debbie had low-stage, low-grade colon cancer, which has a good prognosis. Habib wouldn't give adjuvant chemotherapy, as studies show that adjuvant chemotherapy is beneficial for Dukes' B2 disease, but not for Dukes' B1. Debbie has Dukes' A, which is an even better stage than B1.

I am delighted to hear the wording Dina Habib used. Any doctor can simply say, I will not give you adjuvant chemotherapy. What Dina did was actually explain what the scientific answer is: don't do it. Dina must have taken extra effort for this patient. Your average oncologist sees twenty to twenty-five patients per day. To say "You don't need chemotherapy" takes fifteen seconds. To explain why chemotherapy is inappropriate is a ten-minute conversation.

I am hearing these things, and I am thrilled. This is medicine being practiced the way medicine ought to be practiced. The forces of good got mobilized, and the forces of good did good.

As I hear all this, I think that Debbie is calling me to affirm that she is getting good care. I am ready, indeed eager, to affirm this. But that, I soon discover, is not Debbie's intent at all. She tells me that she has done some reading and knows exactly the studies that Habib was quoting, but has decided that she needs to do everything possible to kill any possible tumor cell left behind.

"I have to be absolutely certain," Debbie says to me. "I have a thirteen-year-old son and a nine-year-old daughter. I have to stay alive for them. I am not—not—taking any chances."

I have some thoughts on this form of reasoning, but decide to keep them to myself, at least for now.

Then she tells me that she returned to Dr. Habib to convince her to give chemo.

"What did Dr. Habib say?"

"Oh, the same thing. That chemo is not called for."

I hear frustration and contempt in Debbie's voice, which makes me wonder whether she is able to accept medical advice that is contrary to what she wants to hear. Could it be that she is unable to take advice from an Arab woman?

"And?" I prompt her, disappointed by the realization that a good story has gone sour.

Habib tells Debbie that she stands to lose more than gain from chemo, that studies show no benefit from chemo in this setting, while the harms are well defined. Then Habib goes through the long list of known harms, concluding with the statement—one that I wholeheartedly agree with—that administering chemotherapy would constitute medical malpractice. In other words, no, no, no, and no!

Habib doesn't bill Debbie for this appointment.

I am still thinking, "This is good, really good."

IN her quest for certainty, Debbie goes to see Hugh Wallace, a well-known physician in the Atlanta area, a socially prominent man who gets a lot of breast-cancer chemotherapy business. Since I don't have much respect for Wallace, his recommendation to Debbie takes me by surprise. It's almost the same as Habib's—minus genetic counseling. On the chemo issue, he agrees 100 percent with Habib. Wallace says that if Debbie insists on the genetic tests, he could arrange them, but the tests would be a waste of time and money.

By this point, I've heard enough to see that the story is getting more ominous.

"So I started crying and begging for adjuvant FOLFOX," Debbie says.

This is shocking. FOLFOX is extremely toxic, which means that you better be sure that the patient stands to benefit from this stuff before you crank up the pump. To start out with, it will cause hair loss, nausea, vomiting, neuropathy, possibly even burning pain in hands and feet. Long-term consequences are even worse: leukemia.

I say nothing.

"Eventually, he saw it my way," Debbie says.

"Are you on FOLFOX now?" I ask.

"Just finished my second course."

I am devastated. Debbie is a candidate for all the known side effects of FOLFOX and none of the benefits. She is also a victim of being well insured and perhaps too sophisticated, but not wise enough.

I realize suddenly that Debbie is the quintessential American consumer of health care. She has reviewed the science, and she has the capacity to understand it. Yet, she chooses to disregard the facts in favor of creating the illusion of control. Debbie is God's gift to crooked and delusional practitioners.

In the 1980s and 1990s, patients like her used to sue the insurers who had the good sense to say that bone marrow transplantation was an unproven therapy for breast cancer. When insurers relented and agreed to pay, all of us chipped in. Costs increased our insurance premiums, but no one paid a higher price than the women whose lives were shortened or ruined by that horrendously toxic therapy. This went on until 1995, until four clinical trials showed that the procedure was not beneficial at best and clearly detrimental at worst.

Where does Debbie get the idea that more is better and that some treatment—any treatment, even toxic treatment—is safer than nothing? Is this idea so firmly implanted in society? Has overtreatment become a feature of our national ideology, a land mine left from a misguided war launched with great fanfare only to fade away from national attention?

We have for so long run on the energy of fighting, beating the cancer, throwing everything at it, that this mentality has overridden common sense and science.

At first, I think that Debbie is rejecting the scientific process and the scientific method. Then I realize that you have to know what the scientific method is in order to reject it. Polo used to say that the word *ignorance* comes from the Latin word *ignarus*. "Gentlemen, it means not knowing what you don't know."

I've seen *ignarus* in patients, and I've seen *ignarus maximus* emerge as the central element in policy debates about health care. It scares me every time. It makes debate impossible. It makes education impossible. It makes communication impossible. All you can do is clash like senseless beasts, and I choose not to.

What can I do now? I want to help Debbie, but how do you find a common language with someone who doesn't believe in the scientific method? What is her reason for calling me now, in the second month of horrible, useless treatment? What is she seeking? Approval or an opportunity to tell the story of what she surely saw as her triumph over the medical profession?

Rarely do I tell a patient what to do. But since Debbie seems to thrive on exceptions, I make one for her. I tell her that she is getting unnecessary treatment and is putting herself at risk. I am the third doctor to tell her this, and I entertain no illusions that my warning would have any impact. I've seen this scenario enough times. Beliefs can't be shaken out once they burrow in. There is no point trying. But I do. I give Debbie the written articles that show that adjuvant FOLFOX helped some people with B2 disease and didn't lower the relapse rate in B1. She has seen those papers, of course.

I give her the science in greater detail. I try to explain, again, what the science says. I explain how we do the science, I give her the actual numbers, I point her to the Kaplan-Meier plot on one of the papers, we talk about five-year disease-free survivals, what her disease-free survival would be without chemotherapy. The chances that the disease would come back are in the range of 5 percent, with no evidence that chemotherapy would push this downward.

This risk of recurrence doesn't balance well against Debbie's increased risk of leukemia, which goes up for fifteen years, peaking at ten to twelve years postchemo. We can't say anything beyond fifteen years because we don't have the data. Immediate side effects are considerable, too. The oxaliplatin component in FOLFOX causes tingling in your fingers, often making it impossible for patients to dress. Shirt buttons are especially a problem. Patients getting oxali are told not to put ice in their mouths. Ice causes burns on their sensitized mucous membranes. The drug 5 fluorouracil, half of FOLFOX, has well-understood toxicity, which includes causing heart attacks. I explain all of this to Debbie.

Debbie sounds happy even when I ask her to list the side effects she is getting: flulike symptoms, neuropathies, numbness and tingling in the hands and feet, nausea, vomiting, hair loss. My mental image of Debbie as a woman with a spectacular mane of curly hair is evidently wrong. The mane, if she had it, is gone.

I understand that Debbie's self-destructive course is set, but I also know that every dose of chemo increases her risk of leukemia and more immediate side effects. Stopping chemo now would limit her exposure. Also, the worse her neuropathies get during six months of chemotherapy, the less recovery she is going to get.

I offer to arrange a formal fourth opinion with a colon-cancer expert at Emory, but Debbie says she isn't interested.

I don't break off the relationship. I get her phone number and ask her to call and update me on her progress. I offer to arrange consults. Debbie calls me four months later to tell me that she has completed the six months of adjuvant chemotherapy. Most of her side effects have resolved, but long-term risks are still there.

I run into Wallace at a local continuing-medical-education meeting and ask him whether he was giving adjuvant chemotherapy to a woman with Dukes' A. The patient's name isn't mentioned, but I fear that we may have violated privacy laws anyway.

Wallace acknowledges having treated a patient like that. "The patient was really insistent," he says. "People like that get what they want. If I hadn't done it, someone else would have."

I can't accept this explanation. It's a classic justification for expensive, bad medical care. It's not different from saying, "If I hadn't sold this person a gram of crack cocaine, somebody else would have."

Wallace says something that sounds ominous: "It's better for her if I give her adjuvant chemo than a lot of other people. I can do it more safely."

Sometimes you hear things that are so shocking that you want time to pause so you can hit a replay button, just to make sure you heard correctly. Is he claiming that he can administer a commonly given regimen with greater safety than any other oncologist in Atlanta? That's absurd.

I know that Debbie was getting enough drugs to produce nausea, vomiting, neuropathy, and, with them, the feeling that she was getting her money's worth. Was Wallace giving her the Full Monty? Was he giving her a half dose of FOLFOX? Was he giving her a quarter dose?

The total cost of six months of chemotherapy would have been about $38,000 plus the antinausea and other supportive care medicines, which can more than double the bill. My friends in private practice tell me that Wallace gets to put about $5,000 into the pocket of his practice just for FOLFOX alone.

Why would Debbie's insurance pay for this abominable care? The answer is simple: the insurance company knows only that Debbie has colon cancer. By law, insurers aren't given the stage of any cancer, which means that they have no way of knowing whether therapy is appropriate.

This is not a good situation: the patient knows the science but chooses to ignore it, the doctor chooses to line his pockets in spite of what he knows, and the insurance company has no access to adequate information.

Could anyone have prevented the harm that was done to Debbie? In a standard small private practice, the answer is no. The only person who stood between Debbie and Wallace was the nurse who administered the chemotherapy. Occasionally, you hear stories of nurses who say, "This is ridiculous," and refuse to carry out orders. To throw this kind of challenge, you have to not mind being unemployed.

The only other check is the courts, which can step in when a patient is sufficiently dissatisfied to file a lawsuit. Alas, the courts, too, have their own peculiar ways of dealing with science and the practice of medicine. Some large oncology practices have instituted quality controls to curtail the irrational practice of medicine. US Oncology, a conglomeration of practices owned by the gigantic health-care company McKesson Corp., requires doctors to enter their diagnoses into the computer system, and if the treatments they choose run counter to established guidelines, they have to justify their decisions. Following that, US Oncology assigns another company doctor to review the justification and sign off on it. This safeguard can't be foolproof, in part because doctors tend to cover for each other, especially when clinical guidelines are broad and when the doctors' objectives include meeting aggressive billing quotas. Still, the requirement surely protects patients from bizarre therapeutic interventions. Since US Oncology treats 17 percent of cancer patients in the United States, it's good to know that these safeguards exist.

At academic hospitals, nurses and pharmacists have more power than at private practices, which allows them to challenge the doctors' orders. Most academic hospitals also require physicians to review the charts of patients handled by their colleagues, to make sure that their standard of care is reasonable. However, that system, too, is vulnerable to abuse. Academic institutions are political, and some doctors are too powerful to challenge. (I believe that bad practitioners in academic institutions do eventually get caught, but it can take a while.)

Alas, the only remedy against a patient who insists on inappropriate care is to just say no. To our detriment, that is exactly what our health-care system is so ill-equipped to do.

Chapter 18

Faith-Based Medicine

WHY DO MY COLLEAGUES IGNORE science? Some do it out of ignorance. Some do it out of greed, some do it out of a weird apathy. This last
group is composed of people who are satisfied with not knowing, with
not being informed. They are not technically ignorant. They know what
they don't know. They know there is something to learn. They just don't
want to learn it.

And who can possibly hold us accountable? Certainly not the consumers who have come to trust doctors, believing naïvely that our medical care is the best in the world.

Recently, at a congressional hearing, I testified alongside a colleague
who threw into his testimony a bunch of statements that anyone who has
taken a beginner's course in epidemiology and biostatistics would have
recognized as nonsense. In one of the most egregious examples, he
claimed that an increase in survival in prostate cancer is evidence of
effectiveness of screening. That's just wrong. Survival measures time that
elapses after diagnosis. By diagnosing a cancer earlier you by definition
increase survival. Alas, you do not necessarily make the patient live
longer. If you have a cancer with a lot of slow-growing and inert tumors,
you can increase the proportion of patients surviving longer than five
years. This is like adding people who do not have cancer to the group.
The more you diagnose, the more you push up survival. To get something meaningful, you have to measure mortality—actual deaths—
from causes related to the disease.

You can explain this to a smart third-grader. But none of the legislators detected the scientific nonsense. I called my colleague on this publicly, as a matter of principle, out of frustration. This didn't resolve the matter, but was taken as a case of experts-disagree-on-an-obscure-point.

The proper study to show that prostate screening saves lives or averts death from prostate cancer is an expensive study that requires time. The National Cancer Institute was doing the study at the time of my testimony, but it had not been completed. Interestingly, a lot of people in the urology community criticized the study. They would ask, why do it when it is obvious that screening saves lives? Eventually, the American study would not show that prostate-cancer screening was beneficial with about ten years of follow-up. A parallel European study with lots of design flaws would suggest a small benefit to screening. However, that study also showed you had to treat forty-eight men to save one life. The pro-screeners criticized every aspect of the American study and praised the European study.

They failed to mention the study showed that forty-seven men would receive useless treatment that impacts quality of life and could actually die in order to save one life. That's a high cost.

Antiscience in urology isn't limited to diagnosis. When treating prostate cancer, urologists are fond of prescribing hormonal treatments. Often, this treatment is prescribed to men who haven't been shown to benefit from this treatment. In some cases, hormones for prostate cancer are just fine. The therapy—gonadotropin-releasing hormone agonists—is approved by the FDA for palliative care of advanced disease. Basically, it can be a reasonable final treatment a man gets for this disease.

Some randomized-trial data show that hormones slightly improve survival for clinically advanced localized disease when combined with radiation therapy. That's not on the label, but it's a reasonable use, too.

These, alas, are the only appropriate uses. No randomized-trial data points to improvement in survival in any other setting. Yet, when we look at patterns of care, we see that one in three men treated for prostate cancer receives these drugs at some point in their disease. This adds up to 60,000 to 70,000 new patients per year. Altogether, at least 250,000 men receive these drugs, paying $800 a month, often for the duration of their lives.

In the absence of scientific data, I can think of only two compelling reasons to prescribe hormones to people who haven't been shown to belong to the groups that stand to benefit from them. One of these reasons is supply, the other, demand.

Demand is where we will begin. It materialized in the 1990s, with the start of screening for prostate cancer with the prostate-specific antigen assay. Men were being diagnosed by the millionss.

Consider a common scenario. A man is diagnosed through PSA and his prostate is taken out. However, after a couple of years, his PSA score begins to rise. He has no symptoms of progressive disease, just a rising lab value. For years, urologists have had powerful incentives to put this gentleman on hormones.

It's logical: prostate cancer is sensitive to hormones; pushing the patient into a hypogonadal state should lower his chances of a recurrence. The result feels like a win-win situation. The treatment knocks down the PSA, the patient is less worried, and the urologist is paid. The problem is, no one can say with certainty whether the patient was helped or harmed. While he might believe that his cancer was detected early and subsequently cured, in reality he could have been rendered impotent and put in diapers unnecessarily and is about to be finished off with a stroke. Is it A (a triumph) or B (a disaster)? No one seems to be interested in testing this intervention in clinical trials.

Through the 1990s, physician-reimbursement policy made administration of hormones profitable to urologists and medical oncologists. Studies show that reimbursement for hormonal treatments accounted for 40 percent of all Medicare payments to some urology practices in the late 1990s. Some of these urologists are well-known, and many are revered by the prostate-cancer-treatment advocacy movement.

Total Medicare costs for this class of drugs in 2000 hovered around $1 billion. At that time, nearly half of all men with prostate cancer were getting one of these drugs. For years, one pharma company gave free "samples" to doctors, who then injected them in patients and billed Medicare. The scheme put several urologists behind bars.

These drugs are rough on patients. Men get hot flashes, headaches, osteoporosis. Worse, there is diabetes and cardiovascular disease, including heart attacks, strokes, and sudden death.

It would have been nice to have ongoing randomized trials of the intervention, perhaps randomizing men to receive the treatment immediately after their PSA starts going up or after they develop actual symptoms. Basically, half the patients would receive treatment for indisputable disease, while the other half would be treated for a rising lab value.

Similar trials were conducted with DES, diethylstilbestrol, about four decades ago. Then, urologists learned that it's better to start treatment after the patient's symptoms show up. Of course, DES was cheap; the new-generation drugs are horrendously expensive. (If money is important, it's better to start sooner and sell more drug.)

A trial with proper informed consent and careful monitoring of adverse events would have been great. Alas, urologists have thwarted all efforts to start such a study. Instead, by giving these drugs without justification to millions of men who may not benefit from them, urologists have staged a frightening societal experiment.

The impact of this societal experiment can now be seen in registries that track cancer statistics. These consequences have been documented in three large registries, a finding that led the US Food and Drug Administration to add a warning to the drugs' labels. Of course, the agency merely urged caution. If urologists and their patients don't want to heed warnings, they don't have to.

To understand the magnitude of this societal experiment, consider another point of information: deaths from prostate cancer have been dropping every year over the past two decades, and this drop has added up to about 30 percent since 1990.

Is cause-specific mortality dropping because doctors are finding earlier-stage disease and treating it effectively? That would be the best-case scenario.

The worst-case scenario is at least equally compelling: widespread use of hormonal agents is causing men to die of cardiovascular disease and diabetes *before* they would ordinarily die of prostate cancer. That's what I suspect is taking place.

If urologists stop prescribing these drugs as widely as they used to, we will see deaths from prostate cancer start to inch up. That could actually be *good* news. Some of the men who would have been killed earlier by strokes and heart attacks caused by hormonal treatments of their asymptomatic disease would now be living long enough to die of their prostate cancer.

Inappropriate use of these drugs can be attributed to the profit motive. A recent study of prescribing patterns demonstrated that as soon as the profit motive weakened, inappropriate prescribing of these drugs dropped. Researchers from the University of Michigan focused on the impact of the decision by Medicare to restrict coverage of hormonal treatments. The changes occurred in 2004 and 2005. How did these changes affect the treatment strategies? To answer this question, the researchers analyzed the Medicare and NCI databases to determine changes in practice patterns that coincided with the change in reimbursement policy.

By going through the data, they identified the men for whom hormonal treatment was appropriate and those for whom it wasn't. Altogether, researchers went through data on 54,925 men who received a diagnosis of incident prostate cancer between 2003 and 2005. They determined that a large number of men whose disease was not appropriate for hormonal therapy nonetheless received it during the era of high reimbursement. However, after Medicare changed its coverage policies, inappropriate usage declined.

The rate of inappropriate use of hormonal treatment dropped from 38.7 percent in 2003 to 30.6 percent in 2004 to 25.7 percent in 2005. This change in Medicare coverage did no harm. Appropriate use of hormones remained the same.

There is no cause for rejoicing. The study suggests that one in four men getting these drugs is getting them inappropriately. The wages of sin have declined, but they are still pretty good.

SOMEWHERE along the way, we have been conditioned to believe that a newer treatment is always a better treatment.

Consider the case of Prilosec, generic name omeprazole, a blockbuster drug for AstraZeneca. The pharmaceutical company marketed it as a treatment for ulcers and gastroesophageal reflux disease. In gastro-esophageal reflux, also known as GERD, the backward flow of acid from the stomach causes heartburn and injury of the esophagus, which is called erosive esophagitis. Prilosec was FDA-approved for these indications in 1989 and, by 1991, was one of the most commonly prescribed drugs in the United States and one of the most profitable drugs in the pharmaceutical industry.

When the patent allowing exclusive production and sale of Prilosec was several years from ending, AstraZeneca executives confronted the inevitable question "What will the next blockbuster be?" How do they keep the money flowing? There was a desperate search for a new drug.

After failing to find their next blockbuster drug, AstraZeneca chemists and lawyers came up with the next best thing. Prilosec was composed of two compounds—left- and right-handed enantiomers of omeprazole. The synthesis of omeprazole created two compounds—both with the same chemical formula, but different. Three-dimensionally, the enantiomers are mirror images, just as humans' left and right hands are mirror images of each other.

Every pill of Prilosec was 50 percent left and 50 percent right. The right-handed structure had little activity as a drug; most activity was in the left-handed enantiomer. The liver converts some of the inactive right-handed structure to the active left-handed structure. Clever chemists at AstraZeneca were able to separate the two isomers and put the active left-handed compound into a new pill, and equally clever patent lawyers at AstraZeneca successfully argued that they should get a new patent for the pill that was only the left-handed enantiomer.

With the new patent, the company conducted a Phase III trial comparing the old omeprazole with the new drug, which was given the generic name esomeprazole. How would you test such a drug? After all, you wouldn't expect it to be better than Prilosec. The company launched a "noninferiority" study, seeking to demonstrate that the new drug was essentially equivalent to its predecessor. This got esomeprazole approved for the same uses as omeprazole.

The AstraZeneca marketing group got on the job. They set out to make the new drug their next billion-dollar blockbuster. They had the chemists formulate the esomeprazole as a "big purple pill." When you set your sights on a blockbuster, names are important, so the company called this Nexium.

The name seems like a jab at us consumers. The company started advertising the big purple pill in a competition against Prilosec. Of course, AstraZeneca marketed both drugs that did the same thing. That Nexium was new and more expensive created, for doctors who don't follow the literature carefully and to patients who watch TV, the perception that Nexium was better than Prilosec. Keep in mind, the clinical trials AstraZeneca presented to the FDA showed the two were equivalent.

AZ marketers began successfully destroying the market for the drug they were about to lose the patent on and converting Prilosec users to Nexium.

Sales of Nexium took off. It would indeed become the next big blockbuster for AstraZeneca. Eventually, Prilosec would be approved for over-the-counter sales, and AstraZeneca would capitalize on this as well.

People who pay their good money to see a doctor want a prescription. They do not want to be told to go buy an over-the-counter drug. The prejudice is that prescription drugs are better than over-the-counter drugs.

Today, Nexium is one of the most commonly used drugs in the United States. The joke is on us. Today, the cost of one dose of prescription Nexium is $6, and over-the-counter Prilosec is about $1. An equivalent generic omeprazol has been available for $.45 a dose since 2006.

I told one of my patients that she should use the generic of Prilosec, that it's as effective as Nexium, but cheaper. She corrected me, explaining that Nexium was new, so it must be better. Besides, her insurance pays for Nexium and it only cost her a $10 copay. I tried to explain that a month of generic omeprazole cost $13 over the counter. Later in the same conversation, she complained that her health insurance cost $18,000 per year.

She seemed to not connect the two.

* * *

SOME of us with a skeptical streak envision corporate chieftains who don't want clinical studies performed. After all, every study carries the risk of demonstrating that your drug is inferior to something else. Worse yet, a study can show that your stuff is worse than nothing at all. Indeed, if you don't look for harm, you don't find harm.

Had Merck refrained from asking too many questions about its drug Vioxx, it would still be on the market. Vioxx (generic name, rofecoxib) was a nonsteroidal anti-inflammatory compound, an inhibitor of the enzyme known as cyclooxygenase-2. There are two cyclooxygenase enzymes. COX-1 inhibition causes platelets to dysfunction and can lead to increased bleeding. COX-2 inhibition relieves pain by preventing prostaglandin production.

COX-2 inhibitors can treat pain from inflammation while not increasing bleeding risk. This is highly desirable, given that most NSAIDs have some COX-1 inhibition, which also has increased risk of gastritis and ulcers.

The giant drug company Merck developed a drug that they called Vioxx as a potential COX-2 inhibitor for the treatment of pain. To get Vioxx FDA-approved for marketing, Merck conducted a series of trials, which might today be considered comparative-effectiveness research. The studies compared the approved arthritis-pain drug naproxen to Vioxx and showed the drugs to be equivalent in both pain control and gastric side effects. The FDA approved Vioxx for relief of pain from rheumatoid arthritis and osteoarthritis, migraine and cluster headaches, as well as menstrual cramps.

In the studies that led to Vioxx's being approved for sale, the group treated with Vioxx had a fourfold higher risk for cardiovascular events than those on naproxen, 0.4 percent versus 0.1 percent. The difference might seem small, but it was statistically significant, meaning that it was probably not a fluke. Why would those taking Vioxx have more heart attacks and strokes? A number of experts, myself included, thought naproxen was preventing cardiovascular disease through its effect on platelets. It was known that aspirin, another nonsteroidal anti-inflammatory, prevented heart disease by decreasing the ability of platelets to form blood clots in arteries of the heart.

Vioxx became a blockbuster. Its 2003 sales were $2.5 billion. It cost $2.50 per pill or $90 per month. While it was on the market, more than 80 million people were prescribed this drug worldwide. Keep in mind that it was FDA-approved because science showed that it was equivalent to $15 a month of naproxen. The only scientifically documented advantage of Vioxx was that it could be administered to most patients once a day, whereas naproxen is generally administered twice a day. It was never even shown that Vioxx was safer in terms of stomach bleeding.

Even though sales of Vioxx were superb, the company was trying to figure out how to squeeze even more sales out of the drug. There was a theory that COX-2 inhibitors would inhibit colon polyp formation. Some polyps are precursors of colon cancer. If Vioxx prevents colon polyps, it might mean it would prevent colon cancer. Another study was conducted. This study randomized adults to Vioxx or placebo. It would have been unethical to test Vioxx versus a placebo in the pain-control studies that got it approved, because drugs such as naproxen can treat pain. But as there is no definite drug to prevent colon polyps, a randomized, placebo-controlled trial in which half the patients would get Vioxx and half would get a placebo was ethically acceptable.

The trial went smoothly until the data safety monitoring committee, a group of experts who get to see the unblended data, noticed a dangerous trend. The Vioxx arm was associated with a four times higher rate of cardiovascular disease and stroke.

An old friend, Bill Anderson, a great doc and a superb epidemiologist, was one of the investigators on the polyp-prevention study. While I was not involved in the public debate about Vioxx, he knew that I was certain that the explanation for the increased number of cardiovascular and stroke events in the Vioxx-versus-naproxen studies was that naproxen was preventing them and not that Vioxx was causing them. He called me one morning and gently told me to start figuring out how the cornstarch in the placebo was preventing heart attacks and strokes.

Of course, it can't. Not in a million years. We clinical researchers call this sort of thing humor. Naturally, Vioxx was to blame for the excess of deaths on the experimentl arm.

Merck ended up withdrawing Vioxx from the market. The lawsuits brought by people claiming harm from Vioxx have so far cost Merck more than $5 billion. We do not know how many people were harmed by Vioxx. Most of them will never employ a lawyer.

A new drug must be better than the old. A new medical device must also be better.

We spend a lot of money on radiologic imaging. The CT, computed tomography; MRI, the magnetic resonance imaging: PET, positron-emission tomography—we love that stuff.

But overuse of radiologic imaging is a major problem in the United States. Up to one-third of radiologic imaging tests are unnecessary. This is a serious problem, not just because these tests are expensive, but because they expose the patient to radiation that can cause cancer. Some have estimated that 1 percent of cancers in the United States are caused by radiation from medical imaging.

Looking at the number of scanners per million population, we have three times as many CT scanners in the United States as in Canada. I am constantly reminding my colleagues not to order a $2,000 CT scan when a $60 chest X-ray will provide the same information. Better yet, a doctor can use a stethoscope to listen to breath sounds in the chest, which is cheap.

Magnetic resonance imagers are even more expensive than CT scanners. They don't give off radiation and are therefore safer than a CT. MRIs use a large magnetic field to provide an image. My favorite MRI story is about a hospital that actually started advertising that they had the only 3-Tesla MRI in the area.

What the hell is a 3-Tesla MRI? For the vast majority of patients needing an imaging study, a 2-Tesla MRI is just as good as a 3-Tesla MRI. Seeking competitive advantage, the hospital had engaged in nonsensical advertising.

In 2008, when adjusted for population size, the United States had five times as many MRI scanners as Canada. In researching this book, I called a physician friend at Princess Margaret Hospital in Toronto to see what the wait time for a CT and an MRI scan was. Then I called the radiology departments at Emory University Hospital and Piedmont

Hospital in Atlanta. The wait was the shortest for both tests at Princess Margaret.

While we may not be able to give Americans the life expectancy that Canadians have (Canada is No. 12 worldwide, with the life expectancy at birth projected at 81.38 years. The United States is No. 50, with the life expectancy of 78.37 years), our excessive number of CT and MRI scanners sure as hell means that we can take more pictures of people dying.

THE da Vinci robot is another expensive device that shows up in commercials and marketing material for numerous hospitals. This machine can be used for heart-valve replacement, hysterectomy, radical prostatectomy, and other surgeries. The incisions are smaller than with a conventional surgery, and theoretically, blood loss, pain, and recovery time should be shorter with a robotic operation. For many operations, more precise cutting is possible without the normal shakiness of the human surgeon's hand.

I got to play with a da Vinci recently. A private hospital had an open house to present information on prostate-cancer screening. They had a demo da Vinci there for patients and curious doctors to play with. It's a cool toy indeed. The doctor has his back to the patient and looks through binoculars to see a three-dimensional image captured by a camera placed through an incision into the patient. The doctor uses controls, like in a video game, to move three rods that extend from the robot connected to surgical instruments. I mastered the art of looking through the scope and lifting pennies with the robot. I realized that anyone who claims to be a robotic surgeon who doesn't look as if he has spent the last ten years playing video games should get extra questioning. You don't want a surgeon with gray hair for this one.

Da Vinci machines cost up to $3 million. The maintenance contract is $500,000 per year. The average cost of disposables is about $1,500 per surgery. Hospitals make up these costs by advertising (another expense) to attract patients looking for new, high-tech, easier treatment.

Free prostate-cancer screening, for example, is a common way of attracting insured patients and paying the mortgage on one of these expensive machines. I mentioned that the advantages of robotic surgery exist—in theory.

This is an important point, as almost all studies comparing robotic to conventional surgery haven't demonstrated significant advantages. Occasionally, a study will show that patients take a few less pain pills. Some defenders of the technology say that the problem is that most surgeons are still learning to use the robots, and the advantages will be seen after surgeons advance on the learning curve. I say maybe. Or maybe not.

Da Vinci is better for some surgeries, compared to an open procedure, but this new technology is being overused and its results are often exaggerated. I worry that we are training a generation of surgeons who may be so dependent on the robot that they will lack the confidence to perform an open procedure when that open procedure is needed.

ANOTHER overused, expensive therapy is intensity-modulated radiation therapy (IMRT). This high-tech treatment is provided by a linear accelerator the size of an SUV—approximately ten feet high and fifteen feet long. The machine alone can cost up to $3 million. The size of the machine usually entails building and construction costs for installation.

IMRT creates a pencil-thin beam of radiation. It allows for fine targeting of the area to be treated. This, in theory, means that less good, healthy tissue near the cancer is damaged as the tumor is radiated.

These machines are being used most extensively to treat cancers of the prostate, head and neck, and the central nervous system. IMRT has also been used to treat breast, thyroid, lung, gastrointestinal, and gynecologic malignancies and certain types of sarcomas. Some patients and some diseases should be treated with IMRT, but most patients with cancer do not need it. Conventional orthovoltage radiation is just as good.

In 1998, IMRT was available at 4 percent of radiation oncology facilities in the United States. By 2003, 38 percent of radiation therapy centers had this technology, and it is available at the majority of centers today. It can cost $60,000 to $80,000 to treat a tumor with IMRT, when the same cancer can be treated with conventional orthovoltage radiation for $10,000 to $12,000.

Some studies show that IMRT is better in treating certain tumors, but it's being used more and more in cancers where studies don't show a benefit to the patient.

PROTON beam therapy is the newest radiation-therapy technology. A machine shoots charged particles called protons, placing radiation into a tumor with no radiation exiting the tumor. The radiation literally stops in the tumor. This creates much less collateral damage to surrounding normal tissues.

This is useful for the treatment of tumors in confined areas with sensitive tissues nearby. For example, brain tumors near the pituitary and hypothalamus are best treated with proton beam therapy. However, proton beam therapy is being used more and more in treatment of diseases in which there is no clear evidence of an advantage. Some are actively trying to prevent studies from being done. Reimbursement for unnecessary proton beam therapy is even better than reimbursement for unnecessary IMRT.

LEGISLATION in 1989 proposed the creation of the Agency for Healthcare Research and Policy. The acronym was unfortunate: AHCRAP. The name was quickly changed to the Agency for Healthcare Policy and Research. (In 1999, the name was changed to the Agency for Healthcare Research and Quality, AHRQ.)

Politicians almost always support basic research, but rarely support studies on the effectiveness of treatment. Yet the leap from interesting science to clinical application is huge, yet difficult and important to pinpoint. AHCPR began with unusually strong bipartisan support. A number of studies demonstrated tremendous variations in medical practice throughout the country and significant inappropriate use of services.

To combat these problems, AHCPR sponsored grants to form Patient Outcomes Research Teams (PORTs), multidisciplinary centers based primarily at university medical schools and schools of public health. The teams were to focus on specific medical problems—appendicitis or heart attacks, for example—and review and synthesize available research, analyze practice variations and patient outcomes using administrative data augmented by primary data collection, disseminate the results, and evaluate the effects of dissemination.

By 1995 AHCPR had dared to examine spinal fusion procedures, one of the great cash cows of medicine, and as a result of venturing into this dangerous territory, the agency nearly lost its funding.

One of the PORTs had published a study reviewing the literature on surgery for low-back pain. It found little evidence to support spinal fusion surgery and noted that such surgery commonly had complications.

The North American Spine Society (NASS), a specialty group, attacked the literature review and the subsequent AHCPR practice guidelines. In a letter published in the journal *Spine* (1994), NASS not only criticized the methods used in the literature review, but expressed concern that the conclusions might be used by insurers to limit the number and types of spinal fusion procedures.

Congressmen Henry Bonilla (R-TX), Gerald Solomon (R-NY), and Joe Barton (R-TX) led the effort in the House to end the agency's funding, claiming, of course, that AHCPR was supporting unsound research and wasting taxpayers' money.

The agency was in serious jeopardy of being abolished just six years after it was formed, but some last-minute political maneuvering secured a reprieve. Representative John Porter (R-IL) and Speaker Newt Gingrich (R-GA) came out in favor of saving the agency. Senator Arlen Specter (R-PA) was chair of the Senate Appropriations Subcommittee on Health. He was lobbied by supporters of the agency as well as its detractors. The eventual House-Senate conference committee decided to cut the AHCPR annual budget by 21 percent.

This story was widely reported in the news media. The spine surgeons were upset that someone would dare to say that bed rest and physical therapy were often more effective than spinal laminectomy. The self-serving surgeons were saying the hell with what the science says, and everyone else was apathetic or worse.

That a federal agency could face a threat of "defunding" and ultimately end up with a catastrophic budget cut as punishment for telling the scientific truth was noticed by those in government. This realization has influenced decisions by officials of the Food and Drug Administration, Centers for Medicare and Medicaid, and others. Shortly after the AHCPR punishment, the National Cancer Institute director, Richard Klausner, was confronted with mammography-screening recommendations for women in their forties. His final decision had to be based not on the science as much as on the politics. Had he pissed off Congress, the NCI would get an AHCPR-like punishment.

His career would be over, too.

Naturally, he caved.

PART IV

Evidence-Based Medicine

Chapter 19

The Denominator

ASK JUST ABOUT anyone you see in the street whether screening for prostate cancer saves lives, and the answer would be yes. "Find it early" is a truth akin to "more is better." It seems obvious that finding cancer early is better than finding it late or not finding it at all. But linear thinking and logical conclusions have time and again gotten us into trouble in medicine. The single most important aspect of clinical research is to identify the fundamental scientific questions.

In prostate cancer, I see three questions that need to be addressed if we are to stop doing harm:

- Does treatment of localized prostate cancer save lives? This question comes first, because if we are unable to improve the prognosis for men with prostate cancer through treatment, early detection would be useless or harmful.
- Which modality is most effective in treating early-stage prostate cancer? Is it radiation therapy or surgical radical prostatectomy?
- Does screening for and identification of early-stage disease save lives? How can we identify the cancers that are a threat to a man's life and need to be treated from those that are not a threat and need to be watched?

Believers in screening have by and large rejected these as legitimate questions and have worked hard to prevent us from answering them in the clinic. Yet, until we know the answers, we will not be able to address the most important question of all:

What's a man to do?

PATIENTS pay doctors to be decisive. "Hell if I know" is not on the menu of answers one expects from a health professional. Yet, every doctor I respect readily acknowledges limits to his or her knowledge. As a profession, we have an even higher duty to recognize what we don't know and ask questions responsibly. Here is how I learned:

In 1989, after six months of training at the NIH Clinical Center, I was rotated to the National Naval Medical Center.

The navy hospital is just across Rockville Pike from NIH, but I would soon learn that the intellectual divide between the two campuses far exceeds the physical distance. Though doctors who ran the navy's cancer program were technically on NCI staff, the intellectual atmosphere they created was more collegial and more conducive to critical examination. These were the doctors who watched with dismay as we were causing paralysis in adrenal-cancer patients.

By the time I cross the road, I have been thoroughly trained and indoctrinated as a soldier in the army of cancer treatment. I have my doubts, but I am still a can-do kind of guy who dispenses hope. One of my first patients is a young black woman with a Dukes' B colon cancer, Stage II disease, with a bulky tumor, but no spread through the lymph nodes. The tumor had been surgically removed.

Since she is so young, I decide to give her the most aggressive treatment available in 1989, 5-FU and levamisole, a drug that is believed to make 5-FU work better. Studies at the time show that 5-FU and levamisole produce better disease-free survival, compared to no treatment, in later-stage disease, Dukes' C colon cancer. If it works in Dukes' C, why shouldn't it work in Dukes' B? This seems logical.

I present the case—and my treatment plan—to the attending. This was my first encounter with Barnett Kramer, a slightly built man who is both intensely knowledgeable and proudly nerdy.

"The data to suggest that 5-FU works in Dukes' B are mighty skimpy. It's really a stretch," Kramer says after hearing my idea.

"I understand that, but this is a young woman, and using chemotherapy to reduce her chances of a recurrence may be a gamble worth
taking," I object.

"This does make sense, but you can actually harm people by using
science that appears to make sense, as opposed to science that has been
proven to be correct in a clinical trial. Worst case, she will get none of the
benefits while suffering the side effects."

I realize that while the warlords across Rockville Pike are trumpeting
therapies and promising cures, Kramer is calmly suggesting that those
same therapies may do harm while doing no good. This is the first example of skepticism I encounter in Bethesda, and it impresses me im-
mensely. This is also the beginning of Otis understanding the value of a
clinical trial and being orthodox to the scientific method.

I want to know more, and over the months that follow, Kramer is
happy to answer questions. These conversations usually take place on
the third floor of Building 10, one of the low buildings adjacent to the
New Deal tower. Sometimes we talk over lunch, joining the navy cancer program's deputy director, Daniel Ihde, and the program's director,
John Minna.

The paucity of our cancer armamentarium is a common subject of
conversations. This is different from the official line you hear across
Rockville Pike: the drugs we have are highly effective. The problem is
reaching "dose density" without killing the patient.

It's not necessarily so, say my new mentors, listing the unproven con-
jectures that go into the belief that more is better. Just as easily, more
can give you higher toxicity without any additional efficacy. More can be
worse.

These guys are particularly effective mentors. Instead of approaching
fellowship as an apprenticeship, wherein the young doctor watches the
attending, they teach you to think for yourself. That trio—particularly
Kramer—move me in the direction of studying the design of clinical
trials.

DURING one of these conversations, Kramer tells me about his intellectual journey. As an academic physician at the University of Florida, he

found himself drawn to trial design and statistics. Early in his career, doctors found effective treatments for childhood leukemia, testicular cancer, and Hodgkin's lymphoma. However, going forward, Kramer doesn't foresee many big cures. What he does see is a need for prevention.

To branch out into that discipline, Kramer attends an intensive weeklong statistics course at Harvard. This only reaffirms his desire to get additional training in trial design and epidemiology. He plans to take a sabbatical at the University of Florida, but Ihde prevails on him to accept a job at Naval. He still plans to pursue a public health degree, but it will have to wait. Meanwhile, Kramer knows enough about the subject to completely transform my thinking about cancer.

Until these conversations, I thought of cancer exclusively as a clinical problem. A clinician deals with one patient at a time, paying no attention to impact on the burden of disease. Now I start thinking of the problem as a simple fraction. As a clinician, I can easily get trapped into focusing exclusively on the numerator—the patient I am taking care of. I pay no attention to the denominator, a population of patients. This distinction is particularly important in screening.

Before you declare a screening test a success, you need to determine how many people you have to screen to detect one instance of disease and how many people you have to screen and treat to save one life. At what point is screening worth the trade-off? What kinds of studies do you need to conduct before you pronounce your test successful?

These questions would change the direction of my career.

Chapter 20

From the Health Fair

SHORTLY AFTER HE TURNS SEVENTY, Ralph DeAngelo, a retired department-store manager, sees a newspaper ad placed by a local Midwestern hospital. The ad says that prostate cancer screening saves lives. It notes that 95 percent of men diagnosed with localized disease are cured. They survive. The ad notes that a local hospital is offering free prostate-cancer screening at a suburban shopping mall during something called Prostate Cancer Awareness Week.

Actually, Ralph isn't the one who notices the ad. He is healthy enough, and he wants to stay that way. Yet, his wife's admonitions notwithstanding, Ralph doesn't frequent doctors' offices. I agree with this approach to life, but Ann DeAngelo doesn't. She loves Ralph, needs him, and this preemptive test for a deadly disease would keep him around for years to come. Ann's reaction to the ad isn't an accident. Campaigns promoting prostate-cancer screening are designed to be noticed by wives, who convince their husbands to get tested.

Ralph doesn't put up a fight. Why would he? He has the time. He is retired. Time isn't scarce. Ralph decides to go, to appease Ann, to stop her worrying, to make her feel more secure about his health, his age, his ability to be there for her. He shows up at the appointed place and waits in line for nearly two hours. The health fair is held in an empty storefront that had been occupied by a succession of five-and-dime stores. It's a maze of partitions, card tables, and balloons. Music of the fifties, and certain kinds of music from the sixties and seventies, create a celebratory feeling.

Guys from a local chapter of a support group called Us TOO International Prostate Cancer Education & Support Network are all around, greeting you, trying to start conversations. The health fair gets men screened and out quickly. It's simple enough. There is no information to take home, no fine print to stumble through, no documents to describe pros and cons. Ralph does fill out a form asking the usual: name, address, date of birth, phone number.

The form doesn't ask for his insurer's name and number, but it does ask whether he is insured and whether he has Medicare and Medicare coinsurance. This seems odd: wasn't this affair billed as a *free* screening? Ralph fills out the forms and waits for his name to be called.

Finally, he steps behind a hospital-blue cloth screen. A urologist in a white coat has him drop his pants and bend over. It's a digital rectal exam. Ralph has had those before. It's just a small indignity that comes with being old. Almost anything is better than the alternative, he thinks as the urologist's index finger draws a sweeping motion inside his rectum.

Ralph rolls up his sleeve to get blood drawn for a test that will measure the level of prostate-specific antigen, or PSA, that famous test that, according to the ad, saves lives. Done. Ralph is free to go on with his life. Ann is officially off his back, appeased.

Two weeks later, a letter from the health system shows up. Ralph's PSA is elevated and he needs to contact a particular office at the hospital. The letter notes that most abnormal PSAs aren't due to cancer. Still, Ralph's test results are significantly abnormal and should be evaluated. Ralph calls the office and gets a referral to a urologist, Philip Moore. Two weeks later is the closest thing they have. Ralph makes the appointment and settles in for the two weeks of hell that follow.

Usually an even-keeled guy, he realizes that he is scared out of his wits. It seems every thought he has begins with cancer or ends with it. Kids and grandkids find out. They, too, worry. Ralph is particularly troubled about some numskull's telling his thirteen-year-old granddaughter. He learns about this the hard way. "Grandpa, are you going to die?" the teary-eyed girl asks him.

Ralph reads up on Moore. The doctor is in his fifties and has been practicing in town for more than twenty-five years. He is part of a five-man group affiliated with a respected local private hospital.

Moore's office is busy. You have to hunt for a chair in the waiting room. Ralph picks up a two-month-old copy of *Field & Stream,* but can't concentrate on the articles or even the pictures. He listens instead. Many guys in the waiting room have abnormal screens that were picked up at the same health fair Ralph attended.

The wait is long, but in the end Ralph gets his twenty minutes with Moore. The doctor examines Ralph's prostate again and prescribes antibiotics in case this PSA elevation is due to prostatitis, a benign inflammation of the prostate. An inflammation can push up your PSA. They will repeat the PSA after several weeks of antibiotics, and if the score is still high, they'll be pretty sure it's prostate cancer.

Ralph was hoping to find out whether he has cancer that very day. After thinking about it for two weeks nonstop, he isn't as afraid of it as one might think. Ralph is ready to duke it out, he's ready to start fighting. Instead, he is faced with more waiting. He stuffs the prescription in his pocket, makes another appointment, and leaves. If the place had a door that could be slammed, he would have slammed it.

Ralph takes the antibiotic religiously. His worry about the Big C is obvious. It affects his relationships with friends and family. He loses interest in family gatherings. His poker buddies notice a change. He thinks about the cancer virtually all the time. He goes to sleep every night envisioning a smoldering fire deep in his pelvis. He is standing face-to-face with the Grim Reaper, staring into his vacant eye sockets.

Ralph returns to Moore and gets blood drawn for a repeat PSA. Twenty-four hours of waiting and praying follow. He finds his mother's rosary, and he prays in his den, with the door closed.

The result comes back at 4.3 ng/ml, 0.3 above what is considered normal. Moore's office assistant tells Ralph over the phone that he needs to come back and get a biopsy. The next available opening is a week later. All added up, it is now six weeks after the original screening at the mall.

The biopsy takes ten minutes and is actually twelve biopsies, six on the left and six on the right. Ralph later recalls that he learned that there is a left and right side of the prostate. He learned by feeling—the biopsies hurt like hell. Ralph is told that it will be three to four days before the results are known.

At the biopsy, for the first time in years, Ralph gets his blood pressure taken. It's high: 160/105. Moore suggests that Ralph see an internist. The internist starts therapy with enalapril, an ACE inhibitor. It works well enough.

Now comes verdict time: Ralph returns to Moore's office, this time with Ann. Things are looking grim, and she has to be in the know. Moore seats them in his office and gives them the news. Two of the twelve biopsies show cancer. They are Gleason 3 plus 3.

This score is associated with the most commonly diagnosed and most commonly treated form of prostate cancer. There is no way to know whether a patient with this diagnosis will develop metastatic disease or live a normal life unaffected by disease. This uncertainty goes back to the way urologists assess and categorize cancer.

The problem is, we still identify cancer optically, classifying tumor cells as they appear in the microscope. It's telling that the founder of that approach—the German scientist Rudolf Virchow—made his principal contributions to science in the mid-nineteenth century. Classifications based on what we see—Virchow actually made drawings—don't always tell us how the disease will behave. Will it turn aggressive or will it sit in place? Does it need to be treated aggressively or should it be left alone? In the case of a Gleason 3 plus 3 tumor, you just don't know.

It would be nice to have molecular-level definitions of prostate and other tumors, but medicine based on genomics and proteomics isn't there yet. Relying on 140-year-old technology, we say to our patients, "There is something here that may or may not kill you."

The two bad biopsies are next to each other in the right side of the prostate. Ten to 15 percent of each of the biopsies has cancer. Ralph and Ann are overwhelmed, yet somehow relieved. They feared this moment for weeks, but hearing the words "You have cancer" brings some resolution. At least they know what they are up against.

Ralph is mostly healthy. He has no history of medical problems, and his moderate hypertension is now well controlled. Moore suggests that Ralph get his prostate surgically removed, a radical prostatectomy. Ralph asks the doctor about side effects.

"Are you still able to have erections?" Moore asks.

Ralph says yes.

The doctor says the operation has a 30 percent risk of impotence and a 15 percent risk of urinary incontinence.

He explains that Ralph will have a catheter in his penis for twelve days and will not be able to drive for about six weeks. Considering the gravity of the situation, the conversation with Moore seems awfully quick, way too brief for Ralph's taste. The doctor seems stingy with information, leaving too many blanks.

Now Ralph has to figure things out for himself, to make his own decisions. His daughter helps him get online and he searches the Net for information on prostate cancer. He truly wants to know more. He finds the Web site of Us TOO, the prostate-cancer support group, and reads virtually every word about prostate-cancer treatment on the site.

Also, he finds information from the National Prostate Cancer Coalition. (This organization would later change its name to Zero: The Project to End Prostate Cancer.) It claims to be giving out unbiased information about screening and treatment. Other sites that Ralph consults include the American Urological Association (a professional group composed of doctors who treat prostate cancer) and the American Cancer Society.

He finds an ad on the Web about cryotherapy, or freezing of the prostate, as a treatment for prostate cancer. Then, quickly, he finds a blogger who writes about his experiences with cryotherapy. The blogger says that this therapy, if done right, by definition freezes the nerves running along the side the prostate. So, again, if done right, the patient will be incontinent and impotent. The blogger attests to this, being both. Ralph concludes that cryotherapy is a slick sales job and rules it out.

All the information Ralph finds gives brief mention to radiation therapy and watchful waiting, a strategy also known as observation therapy. These strategies are interconnected. If you choose watchful waiting and the disease stays in place, you may never have to treat. If it begins to move, you may want to do radiation. To Ralph this sounds like an option for an older man.

After reading everything he can find, Ralph concludes that radical prostatectomy represents the gold standard of care.

The concordance of opinion is remarkable: Ralph wants a radical prostatectomy. His family wants him to have a radical prostatectomy. Moore wants him to have a radical prostatectomy.

ABOUT this time, a Catholic hospital in town launches an ad campaign about its new, less noninvasive treatment for prostate cancer. The ad is built around a picture of a young, handsome urologist, Max Barrish. Barrish uses the da Vinci robot. They look like a fine combination—a young man and his multimillion-dollar robot. It makes Ralph think of the movie *Star Wars*. This duo seems more promising—more up-to-date—than the middle-aged, heavyset, rushed Moore and his knife. The ad notes that hospital time with robotic surgery is lower than with conventional prostatectomy, and that postoperative side effects are lower, too.

Ralph decides to go see this young man and his R2-D2. Ralph gets an appointment within two days and goes with his wife and adult daughter to an office in a building next door to the hospital.

Barrish seems personable, likable. He has gotten Ralph's records from Moore, whom he describes as "a wonderful doctor." Ralph likes that Barrish speaks highly of Moore, a competitor.

"You got me sold on robotic prostatectomy," Ralph says. "But I feel kind of bad about leaving Dr. Moore after everything he has done."

"I am sure Dr. Moore would understand," Barrish assures him. "You are doing what's best for you. The decision is yours."

Barrish gets his office to book an operating room in the hospital and offers a date five days away. Barrish explains the procedure in detail, giving the DeAngelos as much time as they need. He doesn't just address Ralph. He makes eye contact with Mrs. DeAngelo and the couple's daughter.

With the robot, Ralph will receive four small incisions of one inch or less at various places on the abdomen. The abdomen is inflated with a gas. A scope is placed in at the navel to allow a clear view of the internal organs. The other three holes are for the instruments used to remove the prostrate. Barrish shows the DeAngelos pictures of the da Vinci. The surgeon uses video-game-like joysticks to manipulate the arms.

Ralph knows that Barrish went to Henry Ford Hospital in Detroit and studied the procedure under Mani Menon. Menon was the first to introduce the robot in urology and is one of the best-known and most experienced robotic surgeons in the world. Ralph hopes this will give him an edge in getting a good surgery. It gives him some peace.

Ralph gets all the preoperative studies: an EKG and nuclear-medicine scan of his heart two days before the surgery. He meets with the anaesthesiologist the day before the operation. Things seem to be progressing well, but like all patients before surgery, Ralph is nervous. He arrives at the hospital at 5:00 a.m., as instructed, and is brought to the surgical ready room. He sees Barrish around 7:30 a.m. The doctor brings in Ann to see Ralph before the operation. This is a nice, comforting gesture, and it's appreciated.

The operation goes without a hitch, and Ralph is wheeled into the recovery room. He stays in the hospital for two nights. His pain is controlled with Percocet. The catheter running up his penis is a bit annoying, but he lives with it.

The second night after the operation is the first night he goes to sleep without thoughts of the smoldering fire deep in his pelvis. He is discharged with an appointment to see Barrish and talk about his pathology, the analysis of his surgical specimen. This appointment would also allow for a check of the wounds and his Foley catheter.

At the visit, Ralph hears good news. He had a small tumor 5 mm by 5 mm by 6 mm in a moderate-size (50 cc) prostate. The tumor was all in the right side of the prostate and was Gleason 3 plus 3. This means that the tumor didn't appear highly aggressive under the microscope. The outlook is good. Ralph will return in seven days to have the catheter removed.

Over the next week, Ralph feels happy, energized, free. The catheter is removed without a problem.

Unfortunately, Ralph realizes that he is now incontinent. This has to be temporary. Ralph starts trying to do the Kegel exercises in which he has been instructed by one of Barrish's nurses. Three months later, incontinence is still there. No better, no worse. Ralph is wearing diapers continuously. Barrish is reassuring, but there is no improvement.

Before the surgery, Ralph was able to get erections, and he and Ann enjoyed sex. Since getting the news that his PSA was elevated, he has not been able to perform. Could the stress have caused impotence? Or was it the prostate cancer, chipping away?

The doctor who treated his blood pressure gives Ralph a trial pack of Viagra. It does no good. The internist and urologist tell him to be patient as sometimes men can start getting erections six to nine months after surgery.

Soon, Ralph has to confront another calamity: three months after surgery, his PSA is measured at 0.9. Why isn't it zero? His prostate is in a bottle in some pathology lab. He has no prostate tissue. Barrish acknowledges that this is disconcerting, but not unheard-of, and says, "This happens." He suggests that Ralph watch the PSA and do nothing unless it climbs further.

RALPH is more scared than ever. He worries that he has metastatic disease. Everything he has read indicates that cancer that has spread out of the prostate is not curable. Barrish tries to be reassuring, but nothing he can say works.

After consulting with members of Us TOO, the patient support group Ralph first encountered at the health fair, he decides to take matters in his own hands. He goes to see a local radiation oncologist, Joe Salgado. Salgado reviews the data and suggests a repeat PSA.

Ralph is a mental mess as he waits and then goes to see Salgado two days later to get the result: 0.95 ng/ml. They are in Salgado's office when the doctor lets this little factoid fly across the walnut-top desk. He does it without emotion, almost making Ralph feel guilty about being scared to death. But the guilt goes away as quickly as it sets in as Ralph realizes that the surgeon who did his prostatectomy was the only one of that bunch to even try to fake compassion. Or maybe it wasn't fake. Maybe it was the real thing. The other guys aren't even trying.

Salgado tells Ralph to consider two paths. One is to watch the PSA and act if it rises over time. Salgado notes that a residual PSA after surgery is not unusual, especially after a robotic prostatectomy. The other option is to do a ProstaScint scan, a nuclear-medicine test, to see whether they can find prostate cancer. If there is a signal from the pelvis, the doctor would recommend radiation to the pelvis to kill the residual cancer.

It's news to Ralph that a measurable serum PSA after robotic prostatectomy is not unusual. Because of the limit of vision through the scope during the surgery, a small amount of the apex, or lowest part of the prostate, is left behind in robotic operations.

Ralph is emotionally crushed and worried he might still have cancer. Now he really wants radiation therapy to the pelvis to kill all the cancer and rid his body of the problem once and for all.

Salgado is reluctant to irradiate immediately. He orders a CT scan of the pelvis and looks for any evidence of prostate cancer. He performs a ProstaScint scan and finds some PSA uptake in the pelvis. The scan is hard and uncomfortable for Ralph, as he has to stay still for quite a while. Salgado sees a "shadow" there. This could be a residual piece of the prostate. But the test results aren't so bad. There is no sign of disease in the bone, nothing in the lymph nodes.

Ralph is emotionally out of control, growing more and more anxious, reaching the boiling point. Salgado senses his patient's anxiety and frustration and suggests something else to consider: salvage radiation therapy to the pelvis. He doesn't try to sell the treatment, just mentions it as a possibility. He describes this as a shotgun blast to the pelvis in the hopes of killing the cancer that may be there. In technical terms, Ralph would get a radiation dose of 7,000 cGy (cGy is the abbreviation for centigray, which is a unit of radiation energy absorbed) to the prostatic fossa, the area of the pelvis where the prostate used to be.

Ralph likes this. He just can't contemplate that he might have cancer and that it is not being treated. He wants radiation therapy to start immediately.

Salgado tells Ralph that radiation can have significant side effects, and that success is uncertain. Ralph wants radiation and he gets it. About six months after surgery, Salgado starts daily therapy, Monday through Friday, for six weeks. Ralph continues to have impotence and incontinence. Four weeks into the radiation, Ralph sees blood in his stools. This is due to radiation proctitis, radiation damage to the rectum. He continues having incontinence, but also develops a burning sensation upon urination. These symptoms exasperate Ralph. He has growing anxiety and fear. He is depressed.

Ralph ends up stopping his radiation with one week to go. For rectal proctitis he goes to a gastroenterologist, who prescribes steroids in a rectal foam that Ralph has to put up his rectum four times a day.

About three weeks after stopping the radiation, Ralph realizes that when he passes gas, some of it comes out of his urethra. He also senses liquid from his rectum soiling his diaper. Drs. Salgado and Barrish both confirm the diagnosis: Ralph has a rectal fistula into the bladder. There is a hole between Ralph's rectum and his bladder.

After several urinary infections, when the fistula doesn't seem to be healing, Ralph has to see a GI surgeon. He performs a colostomy to keep stool off the inflamed rectum and the hole into the bladder. The next step will be a ureterostomy, a surgery that will bring urine to his abdominal wall and collect it in a bag, just like his bowel movements.

Chapter 21

Behind the Blue Curtain

RALPH CALLS ME one day in 2005. He leaves a message with an administrative assistant that he wants to talk about prostate-cancer screening and treatment. He says he had seen my name in the press and has some questions. I get several calls a week from patients who have questions about prostate-cancer screening. They seek me out because I am an often-quoted, outspoken skeptic.

I view it as part of my mission in life to return every one of these calls.

Ralph says he has read my interview in the online publication PSA Rising, and it's the first time that he has heard that the effectiveness of screening for prostate cancer and its treatment has been questioned. I explain that there is significant controversy, and that I worry that men aren't informed about what is known, what is not known, and what is believed. Ralph asks me to go on.

I tell him that most major organizations that have made statements about prostate-cancer screening have either said they don't recommend it, as it is not proven to save lives, or recommend that men be told of the known and proven harms and the possible benefits before being screened.

Often, people who had been diagnosed through screening believe that their lives have been saved and are grateful to the doctors who have, in fact, harmed them. Ralph seems to be different. Something remarkable is in his voice. He sounds vulnerable, sincere, open to self-examination. During our first conversation, he notes that I have already given him more time than the doctors he paid for advice.

After Ralph tells me his story, I tell him that I should be the one getting billed for our conversation. He laughs. But I am dead serious. I learn a lot every time I talk with a patient who is ready to question the system. Ralph and I end up having at least forty conversations over the following five years.

In our first chat, I explain that ever since screening for prostate cancer was first suggested, prostate-cancer experts have been debating its efficacy. Willet Whitmore, a famous urologist who died of the disease, summarized the quandary this way: "When cure is possible, is it necessary, and when cure is necessary, is it possible?"

Another famous and wise urologist, Paul Schellhammer, who, ironically, also has the disease, said that two kinds of prostate cancer definitely exist, and we hope there are three: "There is the kind of prostate cancer that can be cured, but does not need to be cured; there is the kind of prostate cancer that needs to be cured and cannot be. We all hope there is a kind of prostate cancer that needs to be cured and can be cured."

Treatment can have severe side effects, and we desperately need to find a test that distinguishes a cancer that needs treatment from a cancer that needs observation.

I tell Ralph about a clinical trial I helped design, the Prostate Cancer Prevention Trial (PCPT). The trial was intended to determine whether the drug finasteride has the potential to prevent prostate cancer. It's an interesting question (the answer is yes, sort of), but to me, the most important finding came from follow-up of the group of men who got the placebo.

These were men at average risk of prostate cancer. Until that trial, no one knew how prevalent the disease is in average-risk guys, how likely it is to be detected through PSA, and what the risk of death would be. Us TOO, the urologists, and the Prostate Cancer Coalition thought they knew the answer: "PSA saves lives."

PCPT gave us a very different answer. It told us that the majority of prostate cancers found through screening fall into the category of not needing to be cured if left alone. In that trial, men of median age of sixty-two with a PSA of less than 3.0 were consented and randomized to receive seven years of finasteride or a placebo.

Both groups were screened with PSA annually for seven years, and an abnormal screen led to a biopsy of the prostate. At the end of seven years of screening, those with all normal screens (eight total screens) were biopsied anyway.

The study showed that 14 percent of men in the placebo arm were diagnosed with prostate cancer through screening, and another 14 percent of men in the placebo arm who had seven years of normal screening results were diagnosed with prostate cancer by biopsy. So, PSA screening missed as many cancers as it found.

When the trial began, proponents of screening blasted it, arguing that enrolling men with PSAs of 3.0 or less was trying to prevent prostate cancer in men at low risk for the disease. Yet, the study found that 28 percent of these purportedly low-risk men did indeed have prostate cancer.

I have a friend, Rocky Feuer, who became famous for developing a computer program that uses cancer and population data to estimate risk in a population. His most famous work resulted in the phrase "one in seven women will be diagnosed with breast cancer."

If you plug prostate mortality data into Rocky's program, you come up with the prediction that one in thirty-three men, or 3 percent, will die of prostate cancer. In other words, if a screening practice diagnoses 28 percent of men with prostate cancer when we know that only 3 percent of these men will die of their disease, it's pretty obvious that we are overdiagnosing and overtreating.

"So why is screening so popular?" Ralph asks.

"Many people have been told ever since they were on their mother's knee that finding cancer early and cutting it out is the best therapy for cancer," I say. "I was taught in high school that wise men question what they learn on Mother's knee, and most men are not wise."

People think screening is beneficial, which it can be—for some cancers, in some populations—but not uniformly. For prostate cancer, some large trials are under way to find out if screening is beneficial, but those trials have not been completed. I tell Ralph that I am not convinced that they will be completed.

He asks why I am so pessimistic. I tell him the truth. So many people have decided that screening is beneficial and encourage it that the

American trial designed to measure the PSA test's impact on mortality has been hard to accrue to and hard to run. You can perform a clinical trial—or take part in it—only when you don't know the answers. In this instance, too many men and too many of their doctors believe that they know the answers.

Some men who would be candidates for the study are so upset about prostate cancer that they want to do something. They say it's better to do something—even if it doesn't work—than to let men die of prostate cancer. These well-meaning folks don't understand that screening can be harmful by leading to anxiety and mental anguish over abnormal findings.

Screening can lead to unnecessary treatment that can have its own terrible side effects. These things are proven, whereas the health benefit of screening is only theoretically possible.

The financial benefits of screening for a long chain of medical businesses have been measured almost to a penny. This is a game with a predetermined outcome: everyone but the patient wins.

I tell Ralph about a conversation I had with a marketing guy at a major American cancer center. He explained that they ran free screenings at a local mall every September as part of Prostate Cancer Awareness Month. As I struggled to control my anger, this gentleman explained the business formula:

"First, free screening provides free good publicity for the health system. People really feel good about us, because this is a community service. It will cause women to come to our women's center and men to come to our chest-pain center. It increases almost all our product lines. It's cheap, effective advertising.

"For every thousand men over age fifty who volunteer for free screenings, one hundred and forty-five will have an abnormal screen. Given the demography of the mall, ten of the one hundred and forty-five will have insurance that our health system doesn't take. So, one hundred and thirty-five will come to us to see why they have an abnormal screen. We make up the cost of offering free screening by charging for evaluation of the abnormal screens. About forty to forty-five will have cancer. We hit bingo with them. We know the number who will get radical prostatectomy, the number who will get radiation therapy, the number who will get hormones.

"We know the number who will have incontinence so bad that they will want an artificial urethral sphincter implanted. We even know the number who will not be able to get erections and will want Viagra. We know for how many Viagra won't work. We know how many penile prostheses we will sell."

Realizing that I have been granted an audience with Lucifer, I asked the fundamental question: "How many lives will you save if you screen a thousand men?"

The marketer took his glasses off and looked at me as if I were a fool. "Don't you know, no one knows if this stuff saves lives? I can't give you a number on that."

Ralph is shocked. "You mean it's a big business?"

"Yes," I say. "Unfortunately, it's a big business that's easy to get into because of the prejudice that screening must be beneficial. Consumers—and even many doctors—just don't understand the science and why screening can be a very bad thing. Some choose to stay uninformed. Many actually believe in screening and have no doubts—contrary to the science. Screening is like a religion to them. They believe it—they get screened themselves. If they thought it was purely a scam, they wouldn't get screened."

In one study, 80 percent of male urologists over age fifty reported having chosen to get screened. The same study shows that 50 percent of male internal medicine specialists get prostate-cancer screening. It seems that most urologists have come to believe their own stories, while internists are more skeptical.

Ralph and I start talking about the scam. He asks good questions and I answer bluntly. As a result of our conversations, Ralph ends up understanding prostate cancer and prostate-cancer screening better than most physicians.

We talk about other screening disasters. I tell him about lung-cancer screening with chest X-rays. A number of organizations encouraged it because it found disease at an earlier, more treatable stage. These organizations used false logic to justify screening. This led to increased survival times among those who got screen-detected and still died of lung cancer. These endorsements actually discouraged the completion of the randomized prospective trials that showed that chest X-ray screening at best did not save lives and may well have increased risk of death.

"Those who cannot remember the past are condemned to repeat it," I say, quoting George Santayana.

Ralph asks me about the guys at Us TOO, the pro-screening patient group he first encountered at the health fair. I am well aware of that group and the information it provides. (They know me, too. Hank Porterfield, a leader of Us TOO in the 1990s, had nicknamed me the Prince of Darkness.)

Most of these organizations see the cancer problem as being much simpler than it is and push prostate-cancer research without knowing anything about good research. They tend to gather and relish in the brotherhood and commonality of having cancer. Support is important. I am sure some well-meaning people can be found in these groups, but most just don't get it.

Also, in prostate cancer, patient groups have financial incentives to accept screening as the principal article of faith. Screening sets off the demand for a cascade of services worth billions of dollars to various commercial interests. Patient groups get money from the drug and device companies, and occasionally even hospitals and medical practices, because they push the envelope, making claims so outrageous that even special interests dare not make them. Us TOO, which claims to be the world's largest "grassroots, independent, patient-focused charitable organization" with more than 380 chapters in nine countries, is funded almost completely by the pharmaceutical industry.

Despite getting more than 90 percent of its funding from drug and device companies with an interest in prostate-cancer screening, Us TOO claims to be independent and not beholden to any company. Moreover, it claims to provide unbiased information regarding screening and treatment. If the drug maker Abbott Labs had worked up the audacity to say some of the things Us TOO and Zero say about the Abbott PSA test, the FDA would issue a warning letter and, likely, levy a fine.

I tell Ralph about the business model employed by the National Prostate Cancer Coalition, now called Zero (an organization that has attacked me personally, because I have publicly questioned whether screening and aggressive therapy saves lives). Zero sends its employees to a particular locale, partners with a local cancer-treatment center, enlists some local celebrities, and offers free screening. People found to have abnormalities are steered toward the local cancer-treatment center. That center pays to advertise the screening push and helps Zero get donations.

Most of Zero's budget comes via corporate donations from drug companies and surgical and radiation-treatment-device manufacturers. The group's funders include Amgen, AstraZeneca, Aventis, Cytogen, Merck, Pharmacia, and Pfizer. My personal favorite Zero sponsor is Kimberly-Clark, the maker of Depend undergarments.

Jamie Bearse, a spokesman for Zero, says drug-company funding doesn't create a conflict of interest since prostate-cancer screening saves lives, and that anyone who says otherwise is "misguided." Zero's leader, Skip Lockwood, attacks me regularly because I was once quoted—accurately—as saying, "Prostate-cancer screening and aggressive treatment may save lives, but it definitely sells adult diapers."

A review of Zero's tax filings shows that Lockwood gets paid more to mislead and misinform men than I get paid to tell the truth. I am especially amused by the folks at the American Foundation for Urologic Disease, an offshoot of the American Urological Association. (These organizations seem to change names a lot. They are now referred to as the American Urological Association Foundation.) One of my prized possessions is a letter from Ms. Sandra Vassos, then the group's executive director. She didn't even have the courtesy to write to me directly. She wrote to my boss, explaining that my statements confused patients and kept them from getting screened. She was in essence telling my boss to muzzle me. Ironically, at the same time the AUA itself was saying "Prostate-cancer screening should only be done among well-informed men," a guideline I still consider flawed, both conceptually and grammatically.

AFTER understanding the problem overall, Ralph asks me to examine his case. I agree, and he sends me the entire file—copies of lab reports and operative notes.

Originally, Ralph's slightly elevated PSA of 4.3 ng/ml was most likely due to benign prostatic hyperplasia. It's a swelling of the prostate common in older men. Most likely, it had nothing to do with his cancer.

His biopsies showed a small lesion with a Gleason score of 3 plus 3. This is intermediate disease in terms of aggressiveness. Only two of the twelve biopsies, 10 to 15 percent, had cancer. This information, along with his age, seventy, at diagnosis, pointed to a cancer that many reasonable urologists would at that time have encouraged be watched. Surveillance is an active, not passive, strategy. Many of these patients will never progress.

Today, even more urologists would suggest that a patient like Ralph be watched, as it is more appreciated and accepted that patients in a similar situation don't need aggressive therapy. Indeed, recent data show that 1.3 million American men were needlessly treated for localized prostate cancer from 1986 to 2005.

Ralph got laparoscopic surgery early in the boom in this technology. Today, it seems as if every hospital has bought one of the $3 million da Vinci robots, and everybody advertises having one. Few people know how to use a da Vinci, and it takes more than a hundred operations to truly get comfortable with it.

In my practice, I have seen quite a few men who got a laparoscopic prostatectomy that left a small portion of the prostate behind. The pathologist gets literally a bag of smashed prostate, so he cannot tell if the entire prostate has been removed. The section of the prostate that is left behind can secrete PSA and lead to a low reading in blood tests. If the retained prostate is all benign, the PSA should stay stable. If it's cancer, it will eventually rise in value.

I have refused to treat such patients with hormones or radiation and suggested they be watched. They have left me for doctors who are willing to be more aggressive. I had one patient say to me, "God damn it, I am an American. You cannot tell me I have cancer and we are going to watch it!"

The majority of these men, who are treated with radiation or hormones or both, get no benefit from treatment. They get only the side effects. Radiation side effects include those that Ralph had: proctitis, inflammation and bleeding from the rectum, cystitis, burning on urination and a feeling of urgency, a rectal fistula in which bowels and bladder are connected. The side effects of hormones can be diabetes, cardiac disease, osteoporosis, and muscle loss.

I would have tried to stop Ralph from getting his surgery. I might have suggested repeating the biopsies and verifying the Gleason grade. He had such a small amount of tumor in the biopsy specimen, and what was there was of such low grade, that if he had consulted me after he was operated on, given his stable PSA, I would have encouraged him to be watched rather than radiated.

At the time of his screening, diagnosis, and treatment, Ralph was actually confused by the information he received from the numerous sessions on the Net. Us TOO and Zero increased Ralph's confusion and worry. They tend to make it seem so simple, cut-and-dry, without any questions about what to do.

In this case, both the surgeon and the radiation oncologist got paid. They both likely thought they were doing the right thing. However, these doctors benefited from Ralph's treatment choices. The surgeon made about $2,000 for the surgery, the hospital even more. The radiation oncologist made in excess of $10,000 in professional fees, and the radiation facility got paid even more.

Ralph got the side effects, and his quality of life was destroyed.

DOES treatment of localized prostate cancer save lives?

Ironically, throughout the epidemic of screening and radical prostatectomy in the 1990s, no study was done to show that any treatment of localized prostate cancer actually saved or prolonged lives. Some men, of course, got treated and did well, but would they have done as well or even better with no treatment?

The first studies to show that treatment was beneficial were two radiation therapy studies published in 1997. One study was done in Europe and the other in the United States. Men, in these studies, whose disease was confined to the prostate or just outside the prostate were randomized to receive radiation or radiation with time-limited hormone therapy. The men treated with radiation and hormone therapy as a group did better than those treated with radiation alone.

The only study to show radical prostatectomy to be beneficial was a

Swedish study that randomized a nonscreened population of men with localized prostate cancer to radical prostatectomy or observation therapy and therapy upon progression of disease. After an average of ten years of follow-up, radical prostatectomy showed some advantages. It did save lives, but required eighteen men to be treated to save one life. It is important that the men were not screened, as the follow-up for a screened population would have to be longer to see a difference, and the number needed to be treated to save one life would be greater than eighteen.

An American study, called the Prostate Cancer Intervention versus Observation Study, abbreviated as PIVOT, has randomized primarily older men with localized disease to surgery versus observation therapy. It has had difficulty accruing patients as many doctors actively discourage it. With great difficulty, it ultimately failed to show that immediate treatment was better than observation and treatment if needed.

Which treatment modality—radiation therapy or surgical radical prostatectomy—is most effective?

Three times in the last forty years efforts have been made to randomize men with localized disease to radiation versus radical prostatectomy and to follow them to see which treatment is better. All three trials closed due to lack of accrual. Urologists are the gatekeepers in prostate cancer. They generally make the diagnosis, and urologists have not supported these trials. I have actually heard several say they "know" that surgery is better, even though no data supports this view. This is true prejudice.

From a more cynical point of view, urologists get to bill for prostatectomy or observation therapy. A urologist referring to a radiation oncologist is a urologist forgoing income, and few patients know enough to ask for a referral to a radiation oncologist. I am convinced that most urologists don't consciously think this way, but a conflict of interest exists, and I cannot say what goes on in the subconscious.

DOES screening for early-stage disease save lives?

We know screening *doesn't* save lives for some cancers. The right way to figure out whether a cancer can be treated with lives saved is through a prospective, randomized trial in which one group is screened and another is not. Such studies need tens of thousands of patients and take a long time, a decade or two.

Two such trials were started in the early 1990s to assess prostate-cancer screening. One of them is the Prostate, Lung, Colorectal and Ovarian Cancer Screening Study, or PLCO, sponsored by the U.S. National Cancer Institute. It began in 1992 and randomized seventy-two thousand men to screening or no screening. Societal prejudice toward screening made it difficult to find men who would agree to take a 50 percent chance of being assigned to the group that got no screening. Even after assignment, many men in the no-screening arm got screened, contaminating the results. This has delayed getting an answer. The study's first analysis was published in the spring of 2009, seven years after Ralph was screened. It showed no advantage to screening after a median of nine years of follow-up.

After the study's first results were announced, pro-screening advocates argued that it failed to show that screening saved lives because of the contamination, or screening, in the group that was not to get screened. In essence, the advocates were saying that the study was not reliable because they had successfully sabotaged it.

I believe that the PLCO prostate study is a legitimate first look. Follow-up of the two groups needs to continue. There were 2,820 prostate cancers on the screened arm and 2,322 on the control arm. This indicates that the trial can be viewed as comparing a heavily screened group to a less heavily screened group. Interestingly, overall risk of death was greater in the arm randomized to screening versus that in the control (fifty deaths versus forty-four). That makes one wonder whether treatment brought on through diagnosis of prostate cancer actually kills.

Some of the findings concerning hormonal therapy and increased risk of diabetes, cardiovascular disease, and death are haunting. Some experts have actually suggested that the twenty-year decline in prostate cancer mortality in the United States, which is often used by prostate-cancer advocates as proof screening saves lives, may partially be due to fatal disease from hormones. Treatments resulting from prostate-cancer screening may be leading to a decrease in risk of prostate-cancer death by killing men with diabetes and cardiovascular disease before they can die of prostate cancer.

The second trial that took place in the 1990s, a European trial known under the acronym ERSPC, began as a conglomerate of nine studies in several European countries. Some trials screened men every year, some every two years, one even every four years. Some used the PSA blood test, some used the blood test and a digital rectal examination. One stopped the digital rectal exam six years into the study.

Seven of the nine studies were pooled into an analysis that was advertised as showing that screening decreased risk of death by 20 percent. It's possible that the observation was a fluke. The P value—estimate of statistical validity—in the trial was .04. This is just barely less than .05, the level we consider statistically significant. Anything below that level is classified as statistical noise. Many of the study's peculiarities and methodological flaws could have swung the result toward positivity.

The trial's findings are fascinating. Nonetheless, doctors needed to screen 1,410 men and diagnose and treat forty-eight men to prevent one prostate cancer death. In other words, forty-nine men were likely put in diapers and worse for one of them to be saved. This represents the *best-case* scenario. Even if this ratio is real, I don't find it compelling.

The European trials are supposed to continue, and the findings may grow in statistical significance. Alternatively, the finding could lose its statistical significance.

As a clinical-trials kind of guy, I wonder what happened to the two trials that were not reported. I wonder why the data from seven very different trials was pooled. I am used to seeing such things and would expect each trial to be presented and then what is known as a meta-analysis of the seven trials.

My greatest concern is that most of the trials had control arms that were not actively followed. Some trial participants may not even have known they were in a trial. The screened group, of course, knew they were being screened. This creates a situation in which if the screened group was diagnosed they would be treated in one of the centers running the trial. These centers are staffed by physicians who are interested in prostate cancer, many with specialized training in prostate cancer in the United States. The control group, if diagnosed due to symptoms, was treated in the community. European doctors generally are much less aggressive, and in some cases downright nihilistic, in their treatment of prostate cancer.

The lay media and some medical and advocacy groups have presented the ERSPC as a comparison of a screened group versus an unscreened group. It's not. The ERSPC should be considered a comparison of a group of men who were screened and got American-style prostate cancer treatment if diagnosed versus a group who were not screened and got European-style treatment if diagnosed. It is definitely not a comparison of screening versus nonscreening.

While I am critical of ERSPC and aspects of how it was portrayed in the media, I still think it an important study that suggests something that we are doing in prostate cancer—be it screening and/or some of our modern treatments—is beneficial. It needs to be continued and needs to be watched carefully. All nine studies need to be reported separately and as a collective meta-analysis.

HOW can we identify the cancers that are a threat to a man's life and need to be treated from those that are not a threat and need to be watched?

In the 1990s, many urologists believed that almost all prostate cancers in men under seventy-five needed treatment. The publication of studies that showed that areas with high rates of screening had the same prostate-cancer death rates as areas of low cancer screening suggested that some prostate cancer did not need to be treated.

The Prostate Cancer Prevention Trial discussed earlier proved to many that there can be a diagnosis of cancer that does not kill. Gradually, the prostate-cancer physician community is realizing that some kinds of cancer don't need to be treated.

One problem is that few realize that our definition of prostate cancer was given to us by pathologists in the 1840s in Germany. They used light microscopy and biopsies from patients who had died of prostate cancer that had spread throughout the body. Technology has progressed over the past 160-plus years. Now we can find that pathology localized to the prostate, and we assume that pathology is going to leave the prostate and kill the patient.

Yet sometimes that pathology is genetically programmed to stay in the prostate and never leave during the man's remaining lifetime. We can end up "curing" a patient needlessly. In others, the pathology is genetically programmed to leave the prostate and kill or has already left the prostate. What we need is a 2012 genetic definition of prostate cancer.

WHAT'S a man to do?

I believe that a man should know what we know, what we don't know, and what we believe about prostate cancer. I have been concerned that many patients and physicians have confused what is believed with what is known.

Over the past year since the two randomized trials reported, I have started my screening talks by asking how men would feel about a hypothetical pill: if I had a pill that, taken daily, by men beginning in their fifties would double the risk of a diagnosis of prostate cancer but might decrease risk of death by 20 percent, would you take it?

Because doctors use relative risks and absolutes to their advantage in medical argument, meaning whichever sounds most impressive, I will give the relatives as well.

If the pill definitely doubled lifetime risk of prostate-cancer diagnosis from lifetime risk of 10 percent to lifetime risk of 20 percent, yet might decrease risk of death from 20 percent from a lifetime risk of 3 percent to a lifetime risk of 2.4 percent, would you take it?

I have posed this question a dozen times to several thousand urologists in all. Few are willing to take the pill.

I then give my talk on the principles of prostate-cancer screening and conclude by telling the audience that while we do not have a pill with those efficacy numbers, those same numbers are drawn from the European screening trial for a man who chooses to be screened for ten years. I find it interesting that no one wants to take it as a pill, but everybody pushes an annual blood test with those statistics.

I have long tried to get men to accept reality. It's important to understand that life is a crapshoot. There is risk in all that we do. We do not know that a man diagnosed and treated for prostate cancer benefits from the treatment. We know that some do not because they did not need to be treated or because they die anyway. We hope some benefit in that their lives are saved.

Men who understand the risks and the unknowns and who want to be screened anyway should be screened and not be criticized. Men who don't want to be screened should not be criticized, either.

IT's December 2009, just before Christmas. I get a call from Ralph's daughter. My friend has been taken to the hospital with a fever, she tells me. It's a urinary tract infection. Ralph's daughter and I stay in touch.

Unlike Ralph's many previous infections, this one progresses to sepsis, a widespread bacterial infection in the blood. The battle is lost. On the fifth day of hospitalization, Ralph dies. The death certificate reads that death was caused by a urinary tract infection. It doesn't mention that the urinary tract infection was due to his prostate-cancer treatment and a radiation-induced fistula.

When causes of death are counted for cancer statistics in 2009, Ralph's will not be considered a death due to prostate cancer, even though his death was caused by the cure.

He was seventy-seven.

Chapter 22

False Guidelines

MEDICAL SUBSPECIALTIES HAVE A TOOL for making themselves seem indispensable. It's called *evidence-based practice guidelines*. These weighty words suggest that the patient is getting care based on rigorous science and formulated by luminaries whose judgment is not in the least bit motivated by self-interest.

Almost every medical travesty inflicted on my friend Ralph was based on evidence-based practice guidelines promulgated by medical subspecialties. The only exception was the radiation treatment he received. However bizarre and catastrophic, even that treatment choice was standard enough to warrant Medicare coverage. (It was bad—shameful—but it didn't create legal exposure for the radiation oncologist. No one had the authority to challenge him, no one could stop payment.)

These doctors betrayed the oath and fundamental principle of medicine: *primum non nocere*—first, do no harm. Their actions warrant double contempt because they benefited financially from doing harm.

According to practice guidelines promulgated by urologists, offering Ralph a PSA test represented good medicine. The American Urological Association at that time recommended that screening with the PSA blood test and a digital rectal exam be "offered" to asymptomatic, well-informed men over fifty years of age with a life expectancy of at least ten years.

The word *offer* is important. When a waiter at a party offers you a cold shrimp from a silver tray, you reach for it. When someone you trust—your doctor, or a group of doctors—offers you something that's supposedly in your interest, you accept. That's exactly what happened with Ralph. He was offered screening at a health fair and he accepted.

With screening, you are redistributing risks and benefits across a population. You have to perform a screening test on a certain number of people to detect a certain number of cancers in order to save a life. You may be saving lives, but you accept the notion that you are also hurting people—possibly even killing some with interventions.

For example, recently published results of the National Lung Screening Trial—a $240 million study that compared low-dose helical computed tomography and standard chest X-ray in current and former smokers—found that screening decreases the chance of death by 20 percent. The study, which was conducted by the National Cancer Institute and published in *The New England Journal of Medicine,* found that 53,454 people with the smoking history of at least thirty pack-years had to be screened to save sixty-two lives. The patients were randomized into two groups. Of the people who had abnormal findings in the CT group and went through diagnostic workup, sixteen died within sixty days of getting a follow-up procedure. Of those sixteen, six had no disease.

Thus, follow-up to CT killed as many as sixteen people to save as many as sixty-two. The number of deaths will likely turn out to be a bit higher as a result of radiation risks from CT screening.

At this writing, the guidelines for CT screening are yet to be written, but the general principles that will guide them are well established. A person whose smoking history puts him at high risk may want to gamble on the potential benefits of screening. A person who has never smoked, or a person who grew up in a household of smokers but never smoked herself, or a person who smoked for a short time and quit doesn't have the same risk and doesn't stand to benefit as much as a heavy smoker. For people at lower risk of developing lung cancer, the chances of harm could exceed the chances of benefit.

When it comes to screening, a doctor who says, "Let's err on the side of caution," may actually err on the side of reckless ignorance and grave harm.

* * *

"SAYS who?" is the most important question to ask about a practice guideline. What process was used in formulating the guideline? Did the medical specialty that performs the procedure play a role in formulating the recommendation?

There is no shortage of guidelines out there. Altogether, worldwide, at least three hundred organizations have issued over 2,300 guidelines. For example, in 2011, the National Guideline Clearinghouse listed 555 practice guidelines for managing hypertension. No doubt some of these guidelines are reasonable, and some are self-interested and harmful. Many of these guidelines are commercial documents, yet no one promulgates good practices for their composition, no one rates them, no one regulates them.

"Many people pretend to be guideline makers," says my friend David Ransohoff, author of a classic paper on methods to evaluate screening published by *The New England Journal of Medicine* in 1978. "And there are no checks and balances. It's hard enough for a well-motivated physician to figure out. It's impossible for a civilian to figure out."

When you look deeper at the way guidelines are written, the problem becomes more visible. In 2000, *The Lancet* published an examination of the processes used to prepare 431 guidelines produced by specialty organizations. Altogether, 67 percent of these guidelines didn't describe the participants in the guideline making, 88 percent didn't provide information on how relevant literature was identified, and 82 percent didn't grade the strength of the evidence. Only 5 percent met these three criteria.

"There are so many guidelines, and if they differ, they can't all be right. It's like having several different judicial systems, some of which are not impartial and expert," says Ransohoff, a gastroenterologist, epidemiologist, and cancer-screening researcher at the University of North Carolina. "And these guidelines may render very different decisions. How do you handle that? That's basically what is happening now."

Some medical specialties are well-meaning. Others are cold, calculating, pragmatic. Self-interest, after all, is rational. A doctor has to make a living.

Ransohoff is on a quest to help patients distinguish rational care from nonsense and huckstering. His dream is to convince someone—perhaps a consumer protection group—to take on the monumental task of rating the practice guidelines. So far, he has found no takers. Admittedly, the task he is proposing is enormous, but it can be done—and should be done to prevent future medical disasters.

Ransohoff has a fantasy: he wants doctors to recognize when they are providing good science-based care, and he wants patients to know enough to demand nothing less. I share this fantasy, and as the record shows, I am willing to fight to make it real.

THE U.S. Preventive Services Task Force, an independent panel that advises the U.S. government, is arguably the most rigorous of the guideline-writing groups. The USPSTF developed a detailed, rigorous, explicit, and transparent method to derive guidelines for all medical screening. When you screen, you reshuffle the deck, altering the health risks of the people who go through testing. Some of them could be helped by finding a deadly disease early. Some will be harmed by cascades of medical interventions. Some will be harmed by the mere knowledge of having an abnormal finding. One guiding principle for judging such interventions is that "benefit must be shown to outweigh harm." Another is that strong evidence, such as the results from a randomized, controlled trial, is greatly preferred over weak evidence. The USPSTF process for formulating screening guidelines takes years to complete. This isn't because it's bureaucratic. It's because it's appropriately complicated.

The American Cancer Society guidelines are, for the most part, solid and are getting better. The ACS prostate-screening guideline recognizes that the decision to screen could be appropriate if reached within the doctor-patient relationship. However, the guideline in its current form specifically discourages participation in screening health fairs of the sort that triggered Ralph's cascade of misery.

Most good guideline-writing organizations specifically *exclude* the subspecialties that provide care from membership on the guideline-writing panel. For example, the USPSTF panel deciding on recent recommendations on breast-cancer screening specifically excluded radiologists, the specialists who provide mammography. The objective is to rise above medical politics, self-interest, and self-delusion. Should the person who performs the procedure in question be heard when guidelines are formulated? Absolutely. Should this person be involved in writing the guidelines? Absolutely not.

A doctor who performs mammograms or colonoscopies could be sincere in weighing the evidence. His or her biases don't have to stem from greed. They could come from performing a lot of the same procedures and not being in a position to assess harm.

Many doctors don't know statistics or epidemiology, and all of us have conflicts of interest, maybe just from being enthusiastic about procedures and therapies we were taught to perform in medical training. If you are a urologist and you want to perform a lot of surgery, you can find aggressive guidelines that tell you that it's just the thing to do. After that, you can proudly say, "I am following evidence-based practice guidelines."

If you want to determine overall usefulness of a test such as PSA, you need to perform a comprehensive search of peer-reviewed medical literature. Comprehensive review means going through every single study and grading it all based on strength of evidence.

Could Ralph have learned what he needed by surfing the Internet and reading everything that pops up? The answer is simple: No. You can't figure it out as a patient. It's hard enough to figure it out as a doctor.

A rigorous discipline called quantitative clinical epidemiology has been developed to deal with the development of guidelines. The word *epidemiology* means "upon people." Classical epidemiology taught in schools of public health deals primarily with origins of disease. It poses questions such as "What causes AIDS?" and "Do power lines cause cancer?" Quantitative clinical epidemiology asks questions about diagnosis, prognosis, and response to therapy—things that clinicians need to understand to measure the impact of choices of medical services, such as the cascades that can be set off by an abnormal PSA test.

Clinical epidemiology is about cleansing yourself of prejudice, asking questions broadly, and getting reliable advice from people who have no financial stake in the process. (In this case, urologists have a direct stake in the process, as do radiation oncologists, as do the good folks who make Viagra and Depend.) More than anything else, clinical epidemiology is about being ruthless with evidence as you separate what you know from what you don't know and what you believe.

The USPSTF position on prostate-cancer screening is simple: "Current evidence is insufficient to assess the balance of benefits and harms of the service. Evidence is lacking, of poor quality or conflicting, and the balance of benefits and harms cannot be determined."

It's an honest acknowledgment of uncertainty. The task force recommends against screening for prostate cancer in men age seventy-five years or older.

"Older men, African-American men, and men with a family history of prostate cancer are at increased risk for diagnosis and death from prostate cancer," the USPSTF guideline continues. "Unfortunately, the previously described gaps in the evidence regarding potential benefits of screening also apply to these men."

At this writing, USPSTF is in the process of lowering its letter grade for PSA screening from "I," as in insufficient evidence, to "D," as in don't do it. This battle has just begun. A reader would do well to check the task force Web site, www.preventiveservicestaskforce.org, to see how it comes out. It would be a crying shame if this Web site goes dark.

I helped shape the American Cancer Society's prostate-cancer screening guidelines long before I joined the society. Our first prostate-cancer screening guideline recommended PSA for all men over fifty.

The words of Father Polakowski resonate in the guideline's most recent iteration:

"The American Cancer Society recommends that men make an informed decision with their doctor about whether to be tested for prostate cancer. Research has not yet proven that the potential benefits of testing outweigh the harms of testing and treatment. The American Cancer Society believes that men should not be tested without learning about what we know and don't know about the risks and possible benefits of testing and treatment."

In March 2009, the American Urological Association (AUA) had to alter its guidelines. *The New England Journal of Medicine* had published the results of two studies that showed very different results on PSA screening. A U.S. trial showed that screening doesn't work. A European trial reported a marginally positive result.

Responding to this publication, AUA decided to strengthen its recommendation. Men should now be screened at forty, a full decade earlier than the association recommended previously. This struck me as a non sequitur, given the vastly different interpretation of trial results published in *The New England Journal of Medicine*.

The guideline presented at the AUA 2010 annual meeting states: "The future risk of prostate cancer is closely related to a man's PSA score; a baseline PSA level above the median for age 40 is a strong predictor of prostate cancer. . . . Such testing may not only allow for earlier detection of more curable cancers, but may also allow for more efficient, less frequent testing."

Faced with data demonstrating harm and questionable benefits, the AUA doubled down. The recommendation places U.S. urologists in the position of advocating for the most aggressive screening measures at a time when two of the most important clinical trials of PSA ever done point to the potential for doing harm.

Turning to the list of panel members who drafted the AUA statement, I was puzzled by the outcome. Smart people were involved. Where in the world did that recommendation come from? Looking over the justification, I saw that the recommendation to lower the screening age was based on one small study that focused on diagnosis of cancer.

As their livelihood was threatened, urologists gravitated to a relatively small body of literature that suggests that the PSA at the age of forty is somewhat predictive of whether one is at risk of prostate cancer later on.

I am concerned that adoption of this recommendation will cause a lot of men to be overly concerned that they are at risk for prostate cancer and will ultimately produce personal tragedies akin to Ralph's.

INITIALLY, the impetus for writing guidelines came from academia. The entire endeavor was intended to make medicine more rational. It was, in essence, anticommercial. Yet, in the mid-1990s, commercial interests usurped the language of clinical epidemiology, making it impossible even for an educated person to distinguish a real recommendation based on science from a thinly disguised advertisement for medical services.

Seeing guidelines become the instrument for doing harm is particularly painful to my friend David Ransohoff.

Being a decade older than I, Ransohoff was at the forefront of what amounted to an insurrection of young doctors against the tyranny of venerable professors. In the sixties and seventies, these young rebels started to think of medicine in terms of algorithms while waiting eagerly for computer technology to replace their beloved slide rules, making it possible to model medical decisions and gauge the outcomes of medical interventions.

These doctors sought to change the way medicine was practiced, making it possible to replace intuition and "common sense" with science. The literature they were developing was entirely prescriptive. Their colleagues weren't demanding it, and some thought it was either threatening or absurd. Indeed, how can anyone rely on algorithms—if-then statements—to practice medicine? Are they trying to make doctors into robots? How can algorithms—no matter how advanced—replace a doctor's clinical intuition developed over decades? Even now, doctors are free to ignore science, which they do, wrapping themselves in the language of pseudoscientific guidelines.

Ultimately, to get meaningful, enduring change in the system, we will need to return to the essence of the dreams of these young geeks and make the rest of the medical profession respect evidence.

That's just one aspect of the solution. Yet, change will have to come from below, which can happen when the American people realize that it will take popular action to make doctors practice medicine. Supply would have to meet demand.

Before this can happen, let's consider the evolution of science-based medicine, to enable the reader to distinguish it from medicine of self-interest. After that, we will turn to an example of one patient advocacy group that came to understand the value of evidence-based medicine and started to demand it.

Chapter 23

Algorithms for Judgment

FOR RANSOHOFF, the fundamentals of quantitative clinical epidemiology run deep. He grasped the principles embedded in good guidelines at age five. In 1951, William Ransohoff, his father, started taking David on house calls. The boy would sit in a beat-up, old Chevrolet, waiting for his father to emerge from the house call and present a brief outline of the case. This was a lesson in clinical judgment and understanding evidence.

"Dad would come out and tell me about a patient and say something like 'The patient is having pain, but the real problem is that he is not getting along with a spouse, or that he lost his job,'" Ransohoff recalls. "And Dad would want to understand the real problem and actually try to fix it. Patients like it when doctors give them penicillin for sore throats, and doctors like taking credit for making them better. But patients get better on their own." He thought there was something wrong with this system, and he wanted to know what worked and what didn't.

The Ransohoffs are a German Jewish family that had been producing doctors who practiced in Cincinnati since the early nineteenth century. David was conceived to join this tradition. The elder Ransohoff had training in psychosomatic medicine, a movement in medicine that stressed the mind-body connection. Encountering a patient complaining about a sour stomach, a physician like William Ransohoff will wonder whether this is due to poor diet or a sour marriage. Sometimes, the elder Ransohoff would also see people as a psychiatrist. Instead of rushing to make a diagnosis, he

remained open-minded about what the real problem was, never going beyond evidence.

Where I rely on the guidance of Father Polakowski and his maxim,
Ransohoff stands on his father's shoulders.

A s a medical student, Ransohoff was fascinated to rediscover the question
he encountered while waiting for his father to return from house calls:
what is clinical judgment and how might you teach it to people who are
not doctors? The need to break down clinical judgment into its elements
was urgent. In the late 1960s and 1970s, the country was experiencing a
shortage of doctors, and physician assistants and nurse practitioners were
stepping in to provide care that had traditionally been provided by doctors.

As a med student at Case Western Reserve, Ransohoff became aware
of the work of a faculty researcher, Larry Weed. In the late sixties, Weed
developed a tool called the problem-oriented medical record. His basic
idea was to understand the evidence in an individual patient's history by
breaking it down into four components.

First, the subjective data: what the patient told you.

Second, the objective data: physical examination and laboratory data.
This may be stronger evidence.

Third, assessment: this is where you put the evidence together, syn-
thesizing the subjective and the objective.

Fourth: the treatment plan.

"This was very attractive to me, because it was basically a set of rules
about how to organize evidence: subjective, objective, what's going on
here? What's the differential diagnosis? Have I been broad enough? And
in the plan, how do I narrow down the differential diagnosis?" Ransohoff says.

Organization and rigor were key to cutting through the complexity
and making the right decisions. "One of Larry Weed's cardinal concepts
was never to state a problem at a higher level than you understand it,"
Ransohoff says. "Don't go beyond the evidence. If the problem is stated
as 'chest pain,' don't state it as 'rule out myocardial infarction,' because
that is just one part of a plan, and labeling it that would narrow your

thinking, and you might overlook an aortic dissection, a serious problem that requires specific thinking and tests to find."

In the seventies, doctors interested in medical decision-making started finding each other. Most had an interest in mathematics and a determination to move beyond Weed, sometimes creating quantitative models, such as decision analysis, to understand medical choices and their consequences. Many of these doctors would go on to spectacular careers.

As an intern at Dartmouth, Ransohoff and one of the attendings, Hal Sox, would compete over which of them could be more compulsive in taking care of patients. Sox would later become the head of the US Preventive Services Task Force and, after that, the editor of the *Annals of Internal Medicine*.

As a senior resident, Ransohoff did a rotation in cardiology at Tufts University. By chance, he ran into a cardiologist named Steve Pauker, who was using the quantitative methods of decision analysis, developed at Harvard Business School and MIT, to diagram choices and consequences of medical interventions. Pauker would become the founder of this part of the field of quantitative medical decision-making. Working with Pauker on understanding medical decision-making was a kidney doctor named Jerome Kassirer, who would later become the editor of *The New England Journal of Medicine*. Ransohoff was captivated by this work. It amounted to a dynamic model of decisions his father was describing to him as the two made house calls in Cincinnati.

The discipline of modeling clinical judgment was starting to take shape. However, Ransohoff's medical education was now complete and destiny was calling: he was expected to join the general medicine practice he was conceived and raised to inherit. The problem was, he didn't want to.

Instead, he wanted to pursue his interest in breaking down clinical judgment. Had his mother laid on the guilt, he would likely have joined the practice. Ransohoff realized that he had idealized the relationship between his father and grandfather. True, they had a wonderful practice. They treated university presidents and captains of industry, but in pursuit of social justice they structured the practice to include 15 percent of people who couldn't pay. They were on call twenty-four hours a day, seven days a week, and genuinely thought it was a privilege to work so hard. They were good doctors, but they fought in passive-aggressive ways. On rare occasions when Ransohoff's father left town, his grandfather changed the medications of his patients.

The grandfather, Hiram Weiss, practiced till age ninety and died at age ninety-three. He got an unforgettable eulogy at Hebrew Union College, where he had been the chairman of the board of governors: "No self-respecting Jew in Cincinnati would even think of dying without first consulting Dr. Weiss."

Rather than cause a confrontation—something they studiously avoided in their relationship—David's father and grandfather accepted the myth that David would be joining them in the practice later.

IN 1977, Ransohoff enrolled in the Robert Wood Johnson Clinical Scholars Program at Yale. The program, in its second year, was run by an internist named Alvan R. Feinstein, a wiry, bespectacled, curmudgeonly man. In a photo with Ransohoff's class, Feinstein wears a conservative suit and an Ivy-prep striped tie. He took pride in dressing English while thinking Yiddish. Taking nothing on faith and examining everything, Feinstein was a lunatic-fringe teacher who was brilliant, articulate, and totally ruthless about evidence. He was also famous for Socratic avalanches of questions that would make students and fellows cry.

Ransohoff was happy to learn that Feinstein had written a book on clinical judgment, David's area of interest

None of the eight fellows in Ransohoff's group knew whether they would be able to find jobs, as their chosen field—quantitative clinical epidemiology—was totally out of the mainstream. It was led by three titans: Feinstein, Thomas Chalmers, and Dave Sackett.

Feinstein was writing what would become the fundamental textbook on quantitative clinical epidemiology. Also, he was politicking with the major academic medicine societies to allow clinical epidemiology papers to be presented at their annual meetings, which took place exclusively in May and exclusively in Atlantic City.

Feinstein's vision was to create a science that would generate evidence that can be trusted in making decisions about treating patients *and* making national health policy. (Similar principles should apply whether you are addressing health problems of an individual patient or setting policy for managing a large population of similar patients.)

Feinstein had a love/hate relationship with laboratory science. *Rat-turd grinders* was his term to describe lab scientists. He impregnated that moniker with a surprising amount of complexity. On one level, he was contemptuous of people who studied physiology for its own sake, without regard for application, often with the primary goal of advancing their careers. Important insights were to be gathered by the methods that laboratory people used, but a decision about what's right or wrong for a patient can't be based on lab findings. In a lab, you can develop a test that detects cancer early, but data that would show whether early detection leads to more good than harm has to come from a totally separate field—clinical epidemiology, where you study human beings, not animals or cell lines. Ultimately, you have to perform a clinical trial or some other kind of study in people.

Yet, Feinstein had immense respect for basic scientists because they were rigorous. "We must be like the rat-turd grinders," he would say, and the fellows knew what he meant.

The real world is a surprising place, where diagnosis is not always a benefit. In one of his early classic papers, Dave Sackett found that if you identified people with hypertension, you would trigger an increase in absenteeism in people labeled as hypertensive. If you are labeling people, they may end up missing work, and it's not because the disease is giving them some sort of headaches or heart failure. Most likely, they are missing work because you told them that they are ticking time bombs, and they are scared. The label has a downside.

SOME guys remember the exact spot where the girl of their dreams said yes. Others remember where they were when they got the news that President Kennedy was shot. Ransohoff remembers those landmark events with proper clarity, but he also remembers the exact seat at the Yale medical library where he stumbled upon Dave Sackett's article on rules of evidence for screening. The paper was published in a British medical journal, *The Lancet.* The paper argued that the burden of disease has to be high enough to justify an intervention, that the disease left untreated leads to a bad outcome, and that intervention leads to a better outcome.

"It's simple common sense, but I remember being thrilled by thinking, my God, there are people who are thinking about when it is okay to do screening, when it is okay to do an intervention on a patient," Ransohoff recalls.

Feinstein suggested a topic for Ransohoff's fellowship paper: why not perform an autopsy of a cancer detection test called carcinoembryonic antigen (CEA). This blood test had been purported to be useful in early detection of colon cancer—with almost 100 percent sensitivity and specificity—but was ultimately shown to be no good at detection at all. Ransohoff's paper, which set forth the methods for studying diagnostic tests, was published in *The New England Journal of Medicine* in 1978.

TO the extent possible, the US government makes medical decisions based on science. To get a research grant from the NIH, a scientist has to submit her proposal to a jury of colleagues. To get a drug approved for sale, a company has to provide extensive data from clinical trials.

In 1984, Congress formed the US Preventive Services Task Force to make evidence-based recommendations on a wide range of preventive services. For the next decade, the task force was pretty much the only voice in screening.

The task force spent the first years of its existence deconstructing the standard physical exam, piece by piece. In those days, people did yearly chest X-rays, yearly urinalysis, yearly EKGs. After the task force was done with assessment of whether the tests used were doing more harm than good, the institution of the annual exam was gone.

Each evaluation includes a comprehensive review of evidence— sometimes hundreds of papers—and in some cases lately reviews have included computer modeling.

Now, the task force consists of sixteen members who represent internal medicine, family medicine, behavioral medicine, pediatrics, obstetrics/gynecology, and nursing. Subspecialties that perform tests aren't overlooked. They aren't invited to actually make guidelines because their commercial motivation to sell tests and procedures could cloud their judgment. They are consulted during the process.

The best my friend Ralph could do was listen to conflicting parties or make his own guess. This couldn't possibly serve him well, because the whole purpose of evidence-based medicine is to rise above guesswork. Had Ralph checked the USPSTF recommendations instead of stepping behind a curtain at a shopping mall, he would have found that, at that time, the task force had concluded that there is no evidence to justify routine screening of men under seventy-five, and screening for men over seventy-five is not recommended.

Recently, I heard an interesting word for people diagnosed with cancers of unknown significance: *previvor*, as opposed to *survivor*. We have to accept the fact that we are harming many of these people.

Ralph was past seventy when PSA destroyed his life. When you start screening at forty, the potential for harm is even greater.

Chapter 24

Saying "Enough!"

AS HER BREAST CANCER PROGRESSES and death comes closer, Lilla Romeo suggests to her husband, Tony, that he would make a good patient advocate. She is almost subtle about this, except she mentions it a few times.

Tony says he wants to think about it. He is not ready. "We don't have to do the same stuff," he says. "I can be there to support you and give you my input every now and then . . . I'll tag along and maybe get involved sometimes."

He knows that he is resisting because a good-bye is lurking beneath Lilla's recommendation. She is not being explicit, but it's hard to miss that she is thinking that helping others would help Tony with the search for meaning that will begin in earnest the instant she is gone.

AS options dwindle, Lilla's doctor suggests Avastin. Avastin is not a chemotherapy. It's a biologic agent that seeks to starve the tumor by blocking a protein called VEGF, which is overproduced by cancer cells. VEGF—which stands for vascular endothelial growth factor—is important for the formation of blood vessels. By blocking this supply line, Avastin can deprive the tumor of oxygen it needs to survive.

Avastin, produced by Genentech Inc., an American subsidiary of the Swiss drug maker Roche, is one of the most expensive drugs on the market. In breast cancer, the cost of the drug for the full course of treatment was close to $100,000. That's based on prices that would have been charged to Medicare. The hospital would have charged the insurer a higher price. Avastin is usually used concurrently with a chemotherapy drug called Taxol, generic name paclitaxel, which is derived from the bark of yew trees.

Paclitaxel is a generic and therefore it's cheap. However, Lilla has had a good response to paclitaxel in a more expensive form, Abraxane. Unlike regular paclitaxel, Abraxane doesn't use solvents and doesn't require additional medications to prepare the patient to receive it. The downside is cost.

Effectiveness of this treatment choice is uncertain. Avastin at the time has an "accelerated approval" for breast cancer from the FDA. This is, essentially, a provisional approval, which requires additional studies to determine effectiveness. The randomized trials that had been done up until then were done in a population very different from Lilla. Avastin was found to be effective in patients who had just been diagnosed with metastatic disease, front line. That's where Lilla was in 2000, and in the decade that has elapsed, she has received about a dozen different treatment regimens.

Extrapolating these trial findings to her is a leap of faith. Also, the value of benefits that accrue even to front-line patients is the subject of controversy. The debate is, in part, philosophical. Avastin isn't shown to increase survival. Women who get it live as long as women who didn't. However, one initial study shows that the drug pushes back the time of disease progression. Lilla's disease is already in relentless progression. (Subsequent studies would demonstrate a smaller delay in progression. At this writing, the FDA is seeking to revoke the drug's accelerated approval in breast cancer.)

Of course, Lilla and Tony understand all this. They ran the same literature searches I would have run. "Lilla's doctor had been thinking about it before," Tony says. "If you look at the biological properties, it wasn't totally irrational to think Avastin could possibly work."

Cost doesn't figure in the decision, Tony says. Certainly, the insurance company pays, but even if it balked, the Romeos would have used their own money.

"I can't deny, you get to the point where there are no other options," Tony says. "We thought it's worth a shot. We did it with the understanding that we were really rolling the dice. But the alternative for us at that point was nothing. And we just were not ready for that yet."

Avastin fails Lilla.

As the end nears, the Romeos no longer fear death. They fear death from brain metastases, the crushing blows to identity that precede all else going dark. Lilla has whole-brain radiation to keep brain mets in check long enough for her to die of something else. Luckily, everything else goes first, the lungs, the liver, the whole system.

Lilla dies on June 9, 2010, at sixty-three.

LOSS is a strange animal in 2010. Traces of Lilla, breathing, speaking, are on the Internet. Tony clicks on a seminar at NYU and watches her speak. He does this only once.

He puts the Share men's support group on hiatus. "I don't want to be depressing to the guys," he explains. "It's one thing to be involved in the community, but to facilitate the group of guys who are living with women who are metastatic or in serious stages of disease, I am probably not as reassuring a force as I was, so I am going to opt out of it for a while. It would be tough for me personally, and I certainly would not be an inspiration." It's a blessing that he has a job. (He runs an Internet start-up company.)

Not quite three weeks after Lilla's death, her friends at Share put together a tribute to her and ask Tony whether he would be up to coming. He does. After the meeting, Musa Mayer and Amy Bonoff ask Tony to join them for a chat in the corner. Their suggestion seems logical enough: would Tony be willing to step into Lilla's advisory role at the NCI brain-metastases center?

Tony says he would be interested, in principle, but if he is to do it, it will have to be for the right reason. "Lilla didn't want me doing advocacy as a tribute to her," Tony reflects. "She wanted me to move on and live my life. She was very clear: 'I want you to be happy. I want you to live your life.' But she said all along that this is something you would enjoy and you would add value."

The path to advocacy at Share and other groups that work through a coalition called the National Breast Cancer Coalition lies through Project LEAD, a series of rigorous weeklong courses on basic science and clinical trials. If you work through the NBCC umbrella, you take it for granted that advocacy requires education, which means Project LEAD. It's not a specified requirement, but people like the course and are proud of it. Most of the NBCC leadership as well as the leadership of the grass-roots organizations that work through NBCC have been through it.

Project LEAD has functioned so well for so long—sixteen years—that it's taken for granted. It has graduated about fifteen hundred advocates, almost all of them women with breast cancer.

As an economist, Tony understands statistics and fundamentals of methodology. Basic science, on the other hand, is something he can use.

He decides to take the course and in August 2010 departs for La Jolla.

IN America, disease gets political fast. That's to be expected. It's about money: research funds, medical expenditures, entitlements. What's surprising is the difference between cultures that spring up around diseases. Politics is a part of it, as is diversity of beliefs, intellectual climate, and willingness to question the articles of faith.

The levels of curiosity both on the part of scientists and patients can vary wildly from disease to disease. In part, this variability can be attributed to underlying biology: some diseases are tougher to study, some are less understood. Demographics—who gets the disease—is crucial, too. Compare two cancers of the reproductive system: breast and prostate. In breast cancer, a woman with early disease can be given a choice of treatments and data to help her choose. In prostate cancer, a guy like Ralph has no idea what to do, and I see no signs of emergence of data to guide him.

In breast cancer, the answers emerged largely because of intellectual curiosity of one man, Bernard Fisher, a surgeon at the University of Pittsburgh, who started asking questions about radical mastectomy in the fifties and sixties, testing his hypotheses and finally getting the answers.

The human psyche is interesting. We have always done some things, therefore we criticize anyone who questions the wisdom of doing them. This closed-mindedness and desire to preserve the status quo and avoid change hinders advancement of science. Doctors are bad for this.

The often-told story of the Halsted mastectomy comes to mind. William Stewart Halsted, chair of surgery at Johns Hopkins at the beginning of the twentieth century, described an operation for breast cancer. Taking the breast, including chest-wall muscles over the ribs and going to the third layer of lymph nodes in the armpit (axilla), this "commando" procedure guaranteed the patient would have side effects for the rest of her life. She would have restricted movement and swelling in the arm on the side of the surgery.

This surgery was probably appropriate for women presenting with large breast cancers, as was common in the early 1900s. The operation was performed well into the 1970s in Europe and the 1980s in the United States. Many surgeons questioned its appropriateness for small tumors as early as 1930, but they were shouted down by the surgical mainstream. The operation was described by Halsted, a near god in the minds of most surgeons. He was from Hopkins, after all. Surgeons *round* every morning because the original hospital at Hopkins was round, it was under a dome.

Only in the late 1960s did surgeons Umberto Veronesi in Europe and Fisher in the United States conduct a series of proper studies to show that simply removing the breast, and later a lumpectomy (or simple removal of the breast lump), with radiation therapy was just as effective at controlling the tumor as the Halsted mastectomy.

Women were overtreated and suffered dreadful side effects for years because of a failure to question and, worse yet, the age-old habit of criticizing those who do.

GENUINE public movements begin with conversations. In the case of NBCC, the conversations began in the 1980s, when political groups focused on breast cancer started to form. In part, these groups were rooted in the feminist movement. In part, they were emulating the AIDS movement, an offshoot of the gay rights movement that made AIDS a national emergency.

The breast-cancer movement is all the more interesting because of the role of one book, *Dr. Susan Love's Breast Book,* which was first published in 1990 and is now in its fifth edition. Love, then a surgeon at Dana-Farber Cancer Institute, told a story of a fundamental misunderstanding of breast cancer: that clinical trials demonstrated that radical surgery for breast cancer was powerless to change mortality, and that life-threatening forms of breast cancer, even in their early stages, are systemic diseases that require systemic treatment.

There were breast cancer books before Love's, but hers did something new: it laid out the science comprehensively, in a dispassionate manner, with the sole purpose of helping women make decisions on treatment. Love knew what was going on in breast cancer. She had been practicing at the hotbed of more-is-better, the institution where high-dose chemotherapy with bone marrow transplantation was a bread-and-butter procedure.

She fought it tooth and nail, and when Susan Love gets angry, you know it. Yet, the book is more measured than its author. "The reason I don't say breast-cancer care sucks is you will have less influence," she reflects. "I think there is a fine line if you want to get listened to, of how you lead people to realize there is a problem without completely pulling the rug out from under them of what they are getting right now."

Love was not surprised that the book was well received in Cambridge, Massachusetts, and in Berkeley, California. But, to her surprise, it did well in all states in-between, too. In June 1990, about six hundred women showed up to hear her give a three-hour talk in Salt Lake City.

"In those days, I was going through the treatment options for breast cancer, I was teaching the whole thing: the surgical, the local, the systemic treatment, and it just seemed to be going on forever," she recalls. "It was the middle of the day, the middle of the week, and there were all these middle-aged women there. I was looking for a laugh. I was looking to lighten things up."

So she deadpanned, "We don't know the answers, and I don't know what we have to do to make President Bush wake up and do something about breast cancer. Maybe we should march topless to the White House."

Love was looking for a laugh, and the line still amuses her two decades later. "It was Bush Senior, so the idea of these topless women marching on Bush Senior's White House *was* funny. And they all laughed."

After the talk ended, the middle-aged, middle-class, middle American women, one after another, inquired, "Okay, when is the march? When do we leave?"

This shocked Love. "Suddenly, it hit me that the time was right. I knew about breast-cancer groups in Cambridge and Berkeley, but I thought, 'That's just Cambridge, that's just Berkeley.' But this was something else: Salt Lake City was ready to go. It was time to do something."

Later that week, Love and her partner, surgeon Helen Cooksey, were driving to their cabin in New Hampshire. "I looked over to her and I said the time is here to politicize breast cancer. And I am afraid that this is the right moment for this. And I am in the exact right position to do it. And I gotta do it."

To this Cooksey replied, "I'll never see you again."

LATER that year, in Washington, Love met with Susan Hester, a friend who was setting up a group called Mary-Helen Mautner Project for Lesbians with Cancer. At dinner, they brainstormed the idea of setting up an overarching organization. In those days, Love—who can be disruptive unless she multitasks—carried a stack of three-by-five index cards on which she scribbled notes to herself.

Love saw her role clearly, with a surgeon's precision: "You need somebody who is the catalyst, which is my role. I can see the vision, and I know it's the right time, and I can get the people together. And then you need somebody that's going to run it, which is not my forte at all. You really need a hard-ass. You need somebody who doesn't back down."

Love and Hester spoke with all the groups they could locate, getting the conversation rolling. Then Hester asked a Washington law firm to provide a conference room, and everyone who knew of a breast cancer group or had a list of breast cancer groups started to make calls. The groups were being invited to a meeting.

The organizers had no idea who—if anyone—would show up.

THE word spread through political and peer-counseling groups nationwide. Everyone interested was to meet at a set place at a set time in a small conference room in Washington.

More than a hundred groups showed up.

Many of the women who came forward had led movements before, marching for civil rights, protesting the war in Vietnam. There were also veterans of the women's rights movement, gay rights activists, and a smattering of Israeli peaceniks. For that eclectic bunch, street theater was entertainment, being maced, billy-clubbed, and cuffed was the stuff of fond memories of youth.

Fran Visco, a commercial litigator at a Philadelphia law firm, was one of the women who showed up. As a fifth-grader at a Catholic school, she wanted to be a medical missionary. During the Vietnam War, she volunteered with the Central Committee for Conscientious Objectors. In 1987, at age thirty-nine, as a mother of a fourteen-month-old boy, she was diagnosed with Stage II breast cancer. Two years later, she answered an ad for a support group called the Linda Creed Foundation.

"I don't have the gene that I'm driven to make a lot of money," she says years later. "I have the gene that says I am driven to plague those in power to try to change things for the better, whatever that is."

Visco showed up at the May 1991 breast-cancer meeting in Washington and later was elected the coalition's president. "We wanted to make it a political issue, we wanted to impact the system of research and health care," Visco says. "There were groups doing support, there were groups raising money for research through different avenues. But no one was looking at breast cancer in a systematic, overarching way and saying what needs to change in all of these areas in order to help women."

This small, core group understood something else: strategy.

"You have to know what you want to accomplish—unless you are just interested in getting more money for breast-cancer research," Visco says. "You raise the money and you are done. But that's not what we are interested in. People wanted to march, take out their prostheses, and throw them on the steps of the Capitol. I think it's fine to do that, if you do that to achieve a specific goal. I have no problem with that, but just to do it, it doesn't get you anything except news coverage."

From the start, the coalition focused on three areas: access to care, research, and legislation. To stay focused, they did nothing but breast cancer. No other diseases, no coalitions addressing broader health problems or women's political causes. No sign-on letters.

These people knew how things are wired in Washington, and they knew how these wires could be rearranged. They did what they had to—and in the first battle, they seized the day. In 1993, two years after the Washington meeting, they strong-armed Congress to provide $300 million in new funds for breast-cancer research. That more than tripled the $90 million the NCI was spending before the coalition's appearance.

The biggest share of new money ended up in the medical-research programs of the Department of Defense, where it is given out through a review structure that involves top-notch scientists and breast-cancer advocates, smart people like Fran and Lilla. At this writing, the program has funded $2.1 billion in research.

WHEN she showed up at the Washington meeting in May 1991, Visco knew nothing about breast cancer. She had not read Love's book and had no idea who Love was. Now Visco knows a lot: policy, politics, regulations, epidemiology (both classical and clinical), biostatistics, and basic science. And she is not an exception. At least fifteen hundred people involved in NBCC know big chunks of what she knows, and some know more.

"We want to have a real impact on this disease," says Visco. "We don't want to just get more money for the scientific community and then just let them do what they want with it. We wanted to be able to oversee how the funds are spent and collaborate with scientists to set priorities and design research. To do that, we have to know what we are talking about."

Yet, in 1991, the founders of the coalition had no plans to engage in systematic, rigorous education of advocates. This mission evolved as the group started to adjust to its success.

Perhaps one important moment occurred at one of the early meetings of the board, when epidemiologist and breast-cancer survivor Kay Dickersin saw an old acquaintance, Patricia Barr, a Vermont attorney.

The two met at Bennington College, and Kay, who was two years younger, remembered Pat's role at a teach-in in 1969, at a Moratorium to End the War in Vietnam. These events began on October 15, 1969, and continued on the fifteenth of each month. Kay remembered a campuswide meeting at a big auditorium, with Pat speaking about some aspect of the general strike.

"You can't possibly remember me," Kay started. Indeed, that was the case, Pat was a leader of the antiwar movement and Kay, a freshman.

Even now, in middle age, Pat was as conspicuous as she was on Bennington campus in 1969. At the board meeting, Kay remembers Pat wearing glasses with a superbright aquamarine frame. Pat was clearly not about to let metastatic disease get her down. She would fight it the way she'd protested the war. Now, she was building a grassroots network for the coalition—the first of its kind in cancer—and Kay was there to represent a Baltimore patient group.

That Kay was a top-notch epidemiologist had not yet seemed relevant. Dickersin was the first researcher to describe the publication bias—the tendency to publish positive studies and not publish negative studies. Though she wouldn't understand this until later, Dickersin was at the foundation of *two* important institutions of evidence-based medicine. In her day job, she was working on the Cochrane Collaboration, a worldwide collective of statisticians who pool data from existing sources for meta-analyses.

AT one board meeting in 1993, Visco was startled by something Dickersin said about mammography.

"Wait a minute, I was thirty-nine, a mammogram diagnosed me, do you mean it didn't do me good?" Visco asked.

"Sorry, you might have found it the next day yourself," Dickersin said. Then she launched into an explanation of standards of proof for efficacy of screening. Screening young women before forty would do more harm than good, she said, introducing public-health concepts. You have to think of the denominator—the entire population—and consider the numbers of women you might harm and the costs you would incur in order to save one life.

Dickersin was thirty-four at the time of her diagnosis. No one in his or her right mind would have recommended her to get a mammogram at that age. Indeed, even at age forty, there is room for disagreement. The benefit increases as women age and the harms diminish.

At the same meeting, the group sparred over high-dose chemotherapy with bone marrow transplantation. Several women in the room raised questions about access to the procedure. Some insurers were balking at paying, causing patients to sue for access.

"There is not a shred of evidence to support this," said Love. Any group started by Love would have to be about science.

At that time—as now—debate over mammography focused on women between the ages of forty and forty-nine. Screening for women under forty would do more harm than good, and screening everyone over fifty saves enough lives to make the procedure basically noncontroversial.

In 2009, the US Preventive Services Task Force issued what I think was a poorly worded statement that said that the task force didn't recommend routine screening of women in their forties. The statement added that some women in this age group who are at high risk for breast cancer as well as women who are very concerned about the disease might still want to get screened and should be allowed to do so.

This triggered outrage among ardent supporters of mammography. Having looked at the data, I favor mammography for women in their forties, but I am concerned that mammography has serious shortcomings, and that its power to prevent deaths is often overestimated. The limitations of mammography are rarely discussed. That's unacceptable. Women should be told about the known benefits of mammography as well as its limitations.

Breast cancer mortality rates in the United States have declined by nearly one third over the past twenty years. This is to say that a woman's risk of death from breast cancer today is over 30 percent below where it was in 1990. This decline is due to three factors, including mammography. Improvements in treatment are another factor. Women finding breast masses themselves and getting them evaluated is the third. Twenty years ago, mammography likely contributed more to the drop in mortality than it does today, but there is still a contribution. I think of these three factors the way I think of legs on a three-legged stool. All are important.

Many people are lost in this national debate because it turns on statistics, which are hard for even a statistician to comprehend. Interestingly, almost all experts who have weighed in on this controversy estimate that mammography among women age forty to forty-nine saves lives.

Here is what the controversy is about: The task force estimates that mammography decreases risk of death by 15 percent. The most vociferous screening advocates have done studies suggesting it reduces risk of death by 29 percent.

What do these percentages mean?

There are 23.3 million women aged forty to forty-nine in the United States. Most experts agree that screening all these American women in one year would result in 156,000 callbacks for further evaluation, and ultimately 79,000 would get biopsies. Approximately 32,000 of these women would be diagnosed with breast cancer that year. Eventually, about 8,000 to 9,000 of the 32,000 would die of breast cancer.

Essentially, the task force said that screening 23.3 million women would result in treatment that would save about 1,200 lives. Using estimates of the proponents of mammography, screening could save approximately 2,000 lives. The two groups actually see the data similarly.

Of the 32,000 women who are diagnosed, 23,000 to 24,000 will do well as a result of treatment. Their disease will be arrested or cured. These are women who are often diagnosed through mammographic screening, which is then credited with making the diagnosis. However, in a world without mammography, most of these women could have detected their tumors at an early, curable stage by simply being aware of what their breasts should feel like and palpating an abnormality.

Breast awareness isn't the same as the monthly breast self-examination. Nearly two decades ago, many experts started to realize that teaching a woman to perform a dedicated self-examination of the breasts didn't save lives, but did increase anxiety and the number of breast biopsies performed. In lieu of the monthly self-examination, experts have been encouraging women to be aware of their breasts while bathing and dressing. This is a cursory examination of the breasts daily.

Uncertainty about the quality of mammograms performed in the United States further blurs the picture. Everyone ignores that a large fraction—perhaps more than half—of women in the United States get less-than-optimal-quality mammography. More often than not, the mammographer does not have access to previous mammograms. We need a better test, but satisfaction with and the belief in mammography causes complacency. What we need is more support for research aimed at finding a better test.

As we argue over screening in the age group where we can at best save two thousand lives per year, we seem to ignore that 40 percent of women in their fifties and sixties don't get mammography. This represents more than five thousand lives per year that could be saved through simply getting people adequate care.

Chapter 25

Project LEAD

IN PART because of her expertise—but also because she lived close to Washington—Dickersin was frequently called on to show up on Capitol Hill. In the early days of the coalition, only one other member of the board—Love—understood science. Alas, she was chronically overscheduled. Dickersin wanted to spread out the responsibility of talking with congressional staff members.

"I am going to suggest something," Dickersin said at one of the early board meetings. "We'll do a teach-in, just like we did in the Vietnam era."

Everyone at the table could be presumed to be a Vietnam protester, including Kay's teach-in instructor from the 1969 moratorium, who sat across from her at the table.

Visco remembers that discussion. "Kay Dickersin said, 'If we want to influence NIH, if we want to influence science, all of us need to know what we are talking about.' And that certainly resonated with me. When you are a trial lawyer, you don't walk into that courtroom, you don't walk into any argument or deposition, unless you know everything.

"You have to know the strengths, the weaknesses, you have to understand it all. I knew when I was practicing law that if my client had a business that made windows, I had to learn about that. Now I had to learn science."

The first teach-in, conducted in conjunction with a board meeting, was on basic science. After the second teach-in, on epidemiology and biostatistics, the board was asked to hear a presentation by a drug-company executive. The slides included "median survival time" on the drug in question, compared with placebo.

"Median survival means that this is how long patients lived on average," he said.

One of the women who had just gone through a daylong course on epi-bio raised her hand. "No, it doesn't," she said. "Median is not the same as mean."

Indeed, median survival is the point where half the patients have died and the other half live longer. Mean is the same as average.

The drug-company executive acknowledged the screwup—how can you not?—then showed a slide with two curves separating. He noted that some patients were found ineligible and were excluded from analysis.

One of the members raised her hand. "Wait a minute, you mean you didn't perform intention-to-treat analysis? You are introducing a bias." Indeed, excluding patients after they have been assigned to groups potentially allows you to cherry-pick and is therefore verboten in good clinical trials.

"They really got it," said Dickersin. "It was so cool for me as a teacher."

At the end, Pat Barr turned to Kay Dickersin, saying, "We must take this on the road." Kay agreed.

THEY did, ultimately developing a core curriculum and a group of teachers—all of them top-notch scientists—who go on the road with the project. The first session was held in 1995, and starting in 1998, they have been held four times a year. The curriculum has changed over time, sometimes to reflect new science, and sometimes to add new areas of emphasis.

Teachers don't get to bring their own slides; the slides are provided. Uttering a sentence like "I tell my patients . . ." will bring on a talking-to. Stick to the evidence, Doctor, thank you very much.

The course is designed to push the patients outside their experience, beyond their cancer, to the heights where science and policy soar side by side.

Every now and then, other patient groups inquire about adopting Project LEAD, even licensing it. They get a firm no. Even ripping off a syllabus and the slides, you will not end up with anything even close to Project LEAD. To produce Project LEAD, you need skepticism and a cadre of tough, dedicated people who safeguard it. "You need a culture," says Love.

Graduates of Project LEAD get to do some amazing stuff. Working alongside scientists, they review grants for the National Institutes of Health and the Department of Defense. They sit on institutional review boards that monitor ethics of clinical trials. They sit on data and safety-monitoring boards that decide whether clinical trials have met their objectives and whether they should continue. Also, they offer guidance to pharmaceutical companies as they develop drugs and to the Food and Drug Administration as it decides whether drugs merit marketing approval.

Sure, patients who haven't done Project LEAD do some of those things, too, but a Project LEAD credential means that you are dealing with someone who understands the fundamentals. Some Project LEAD graduates are dazzling. For example, Ransohoff can't get himself to delete his correspondence with Share's Helen Schiff.

"I've got a bunch of detailed e-mails going back five years, dealing with a broad range of topics," he said recently. "The detail of her interest is really striking for a civilian. Most physicians don't know half of what she knows about clinical-research methodology and clinical trials."

ALL NBCC events begin with a moment of silence in honor of an advocate who died of breast cancer. Every board meeting, every advocacy conference, every scientific-consensus meeting, and every Project LEAD starts in exactly the same way. A picture of an advocate is projected on a screen and her story is told.

The 2010 Project LEAD in La Jolla began with Fran Visco's tribute to Lilla Romeo. Tony knew it was coming. He had been asked in advance, and he provided the picture.

It was a good thing, though it hurt like hell, or because it did. "Lilla had died two months before," Tony recalls. "I was not at my most raw state, but not that far along in the mourning process."

Then, breaking the silence, Fran simply moved on to her introductory talk. The juxtaposition was powerful.

"Here was the emotion—here is the people connection that advocacy is all about—and then Fran is off and running, talking about evidence-based medicine," Tony says. "We recognize that this is about lives, about people who struggle with that disease. Now let's get down to business. Not losing sight of the personal element, but also getting into hard thinking that's required for advocacy to be effective."

Fran often reminds advocates that true advocacy is about learning from your experience and rising above it. The science at Project LEAD was stimulating enough, but Tony experienced a second track also, which ran privately, entirely inside his skull. It seemed to be akin to a health-care economics conference for one attendee, a rigorous examination of decisions that had been made in Lilla's care.

The hemoglobin-building drugs were an information problem. Lilla got most of these drugs without the benefit of being asked or a discussion of pros and cons. When the questionnaire was finally administered, it was disingenuous, an obfuscation. And, of course, no one bothered to mention the system of incentives at play. The system was manipulating information to protect itself. "I wish we had known that, because I wonder whether it stimulated the tumor growth, and I know Lilla wondered about that," Tony said.

The reexamination of the Avastin decision was more intriguing, especially in the context of Project LEAD. It pitted the private decision against the concept of overall public good, micro versus macro. In his private space, Tony-the-economist was debating Tony-the-husband.

"Project LEAD raises your consciousness," he said. "It does cause you to do self-examination. If we say that one thing is the right way to do it for society, shouldn't we be applying it to our personal decisions? For me, this is interesting, because you don't want to be a hypocrite. I don't want people to say to me, 'You talk like an economist about this stuff, but when it came to the crunch, your wife took Avastin.'

"Was that irrational?

"I don't know.

"I look back at some of that and think we probably shouldn't have done that. But the key part about it is that it certainly didn't help. If there had been a system that made it more difficult, it would not have done her any harm."

AT the end of Project LEAD, students are asked what they will do with their knowledge. This question stumped Lilla Romeo when she first took the course in the spring of 2007, but ultimately she found a great use for her knowledge. Taking the course in August 2010, Tony Romeo, too, wasn't quite certain. He was still thinking about it a month later, when we talked.

"I don't want it to be about Lilla's cancer," he said. "That may have been the thing that awakened us to the issues, but I don't want it to be the thing that drives this throughout."

Lilla was interested in brain metastases in part because of her diagnosis. Should Tony be interested in the same?

"I am moving along in my mourning process, and I need to be doing things for the right reasons," he said. "I am also thinking about applying what I know outside breast cancer."

NBCC stays effective by staying focused. Sure, the problems in health care are vast, but so far they have produced few fiercely independent, uncorrupted, genuine public movements.

In AIDS, some groups pursue evidence-based medicine, and in cancer, there is NBCC. It's notable that in 1996, urologists attempted to build a nationwide coalition of grassroots organizations. They did so by having the American Federation of Urologic Disease, their in-house patient group, secure a grant from the drug company Zeneca to transport guys over to Houston. No drug company paid for the 1991 meeting of breast-cancer groups.

"The problem is, people don't realize they are not getting good-quality care," says Love. "So the first step is to show them. And that's really hard, because when it's you, it's too scary to think you are not getting good-quality care. Even if somebody gives you a cogent intellectual argument, when you are sick, you have to believe you are getting good-quality care."

This is a battle that needs to be fought.

Epilogue

AMERICAN HEALTH CARE has some genuine successes.

Recently, I met a twelve-year-old girl named Grace. She is a cancer survivor, cured of neuroblastoma several years ago. Grace was a thriving seventeen-month-old toddler living in Paducah, Kentucky, when she developed swelling and a bruised appearance around her right eye. The pediatrician initially thought it a black eye from some trauma. When it did not improve over several days, the doctor did a more thorough examination and suspected the liver was enlarged or a mass was in the abdomen.

An ultrasound of the abdomen showed a mass in the adrenal gland and liver. Ultrasound of the eye orbit was nondiagnostic. Magnetic resonance imaging of the head was done with anaesthesia, to keep Grace from moving. A mass was infiltrating the bones about the right eye and extended into the sella. The sella is the part of the skull at the base of the brain where the hypothalamus and pituitary gland are located.

The pediatrician referred Grace to the Cincinnati Children's Hospital. She explained to Grace's concerned parents that this was serious. Grace almost certainly had a cancer, and it had spread. It was in her head and abdomen. Her eye and her liver and adrenal gland were clearly affected. Other organs might be involved. A biopsy needed to be done to determine what this was.

The parents asked about prognosis. The pediatrician said she could not say. Anything she said would be a guess. This could be a lymphoma, which meant a possibility of a cure. It could also be an incurable cancer.

Years later, Grace's mom still talks about how the four days' wait to see the pediatricians at the Cincinnati Children's Hospital seemed like an eternity. The five-hour drive to Cincinnati seemed never ending.

At the hospital, the family met with a group of pediatric oncologists and a group of nurses and social workers. The mass in the abdomen involved the adrenal and the liver, but could be surgically removed. This operation would allow the surgeons to get tissue and determine a diagnosis. Surgery was scheduled for three days later. The child was admitted to the hospital and began a regimen to clean out her bowels in case the pediatric surgeon needed to cut into the bowel. This was the start of a six-month ordeal of therapy.

Grace was diagnosed early in the Internet age, but her parents learned a great deal about neuroblastoma and its treatment on the Web, allowing them to figure out what questions they needed to ask.

Grace was fortunate. She had interested parents who remained objective and focused without panic. One can be emotional and care without panic. Grace had good doctors and health-care providers (nurses, social workers) at every stage of her therapy. They knew what to do and were good at explaining it and supporting the patient and her parents. Her treatment involved the appropriate use of surgery in her abdomen, high-dose chemotherapy, and high-tech proton-beam radiation therapy to the eye and base of brain.

Grace did well because she got the right therapy. In the United States, pediatric oncology is generally well organized and seems to treat patients at a consistently higher standard than we in adult medicine do. We don't hear about pediatric oncologists providing unnecessary therapy, as we do among adults. I often think that pediatric medicine attracts people who are good human beings who care—folks who realize that being a professional means you put the well-being of your patients above your own well-being.

America is a great place to get health care if you can afford it and if you are fortunate enough to know my friend Al Rabson or someone else who can help you get to good doctors.

Grace also had insurance. Insurance is important if you are to get good health care. Now, Grace is free of neuroblastoma, but her treatment puts her at increased risk of eventually developing leukemia. Kids who survive cancer often have side effects from therapy. Stunted growth, decreased mental abilities, constant worry, and post-traumatic stress disorder are all problems of childhood-cancer survivors. Prior to the enactment of recent health-care reform legislation, kids who survived cancer were often unable to get health insurance due to preexisting conditions.

ALAS, wealth can also steer a person toward bad doctors. Some wealthy patients have to have the chair of the department as their doctor, or to go to the society doctor. These doctors practice the best of medicine of the year they graduated from medical school.

Consider the case of an academic physician who had been known to get his doses wrong. Physician practices at academic institutions routinely have doctors review each other's charts. This doctor appeared to prescribe unusual treatments and make mistakes in the calculation of doses. Even when administered properly, cancer drugs can bring the patient to the brink of death. An overdose can easily push him off the cliff.

The problem hadn't reached the level where the doctor could be fired; or, for reasons that may at least in part have been political, dismissal was not an option. Besides, dismissal, like disease, is a process. It has to play out. The findings were bad enough to cause the institution to place this physician under intensive monitoring. Every order this individual wrote had to be cosigned by another doctor and a pharmacist.

This doctor had a hunch that a regimen he had devised would be effective in the treatment of triple-negative breast cancer. His regimen included an old chemotherapy drug that hadn't been used in oral form for at least a quarter century. The idea was intriguing: instead of giving a drug intravenously every three weeks, why not give it orally every day for two weeks? Instead of zapping the patient with a large amount of the agent and having it wash out fast, you let it build up slowly.

Nothing is wrong with experimentation as long as you write a protocol, get it approved, obtain consent from your subjects, and submit to oversight by an institutional review board. In this case, the doctor apparently decided to test out the lab findings by staging an experiment on one patient.

However, this physician was already under review, and the reviewer and the pharmacist would never sign off on an oddball regimen. To bypass them, the physician wrote a prescription, and the patient had it filled at a local pharmacy. The pharmacist, who wasn't used to dispensing cancer drugs, even in oral form, saw no problem, and the doctor effectively skirted institutional oversight.

Calculation of the dose was a problem, though. Usually, a 120-pound woman would get 120 milligrams of the oral version of the drug daily. If the drug is infused intravenously, she would get 720 milligrams— six times as much—every three weeks. The doctor apparently got things confused and prescribed the oral drug in what would have been a reasonable IV dose. Had the patient completed the prescribed course of treatment, she would have ended up receiving a cumulative dose that would have been eighty-four times the amount that would have been standard.

The patient never finished the entire course. She developed a severe suppression of white blood cells and a fever and was hospitalized. Fortunately, she survived. The doctor in question was confronted, and ultimately a deal was reached: the doctor agreed to surrender his clinical privileges, and in exchange, the institution agreed not to press for the removal of this doctor's license to practice medicine.

This means that in the future this doctor may be practicing medicine somewhere else, perhaps even dosing you or someone you know.

I know of one line of defense against these dangerous luminaries: challenge them to justify their treatment decisions.

LILLA and Tony Romeo are probably the most sophisticated health-care consumers you will ever meet, yet even they were powerless to protect themselves from red juice. And we chipped in, because their insurer failed to ask tough questions that were becoming increasingly obvious.

The system is not failing. It's functioning exactly as designed. It's designed to run up health-care costs. It's about the greedy serving the gluttonous. Americans consume more health care per capita than the people of any other country. In 2009, we spent more than $2.53 trillion. That's 2.5 times more than we spent on food. It's not easy to envision a trillion. Let's fix that:

A million seconds was twelve days ago. A billion seconds was thirty-two years ago. A trillion seconds was 30,000 years BCE.

We desperately need to focus on rational consumption of health care. Rational consumption includes preventive services and health education. Much of the money currently spent on health care is money wasted on unnecessary and harmful, sick care. Even for the sick, a lot of necessary care is not given at the appropriate time. The result is more expensive care given later.

A rational system would stress prevention and health education. We could use a lot of that. In 1970, 4 percent of American kids, aged five to eleven, were obese; today, more than 20 percent are. In 1970, 15 percent of American adults were obese; today, more than 35 percent are. This uniquely American obesity epidemic is causing a rise in the rates of a number of chronic diseases. The prevalence of diabetes, cardiovascular disease, stroke, orthopedic injury, and cancer are all affected by obesity, high caloric intake, and lack of exercise. Consumption of medical care and health-care costs are destined to grow dramatically due to this tsunami of chronic disease.

Waste in medicine could be reduced if only we were more rational. The bad actors include doctors and health-care providers, hospitals, drug and device manufacturers, insurance companies, lawyers, and patients. If Polo were alive today, he would say that three evils have infected American medicine: apathy, ignorance, and greed.

The 51 million American adults who have no insurance live desperate lives. The system almost certainly killed Cedric Jones by denying him the defibrillator he needed. But even those who have insurance can be excluded from care. Edna Riggs was—at least in the beginning—insured.

Some of the apathetic are those who are satisfied with the health-care system and perceive that they have access. Many of those people will be surprised to learn that their health insurance is not as good as they thought it was. Helen Williams was getting what she thought was the best care imaginable while we were paying for her unproven, abominable care. Martin Schmidt was insured, too.

Some of the apathetic are those like the lady who wants a prescription for Nexium and notes that her insurance pays for it. She doesn't want the cheaper equivalent, Prilosec. If you are willing to pay twelve times more than you need to for the privilege of taking Nexium, you are not being patriotic, you are not being a patron of science, and you are not earning the respect of the drug's maker. As a scientist, I can assure you that we are being laughed at.

The rich and the insured should not be protected from their own folly. They should not be subsidized as they make decisions that are akin to those of the Huzjak children. Debbie Kurtz should not be shielded from the financial consequences of getting the unjustifiable care that presumably helped an unscrupulous doctor make a payment on a Mercedes. The Mercedes dealership should probably send thank-you notes to everyone who pays premiums to the insurance company that wrote Debbie's policy. She may still pay for her foolishness by getting leukemia later in life.

The medical profession frequently allows bad doctors to continue to practice. The profession doesn't police itself. Chalk it up to apathy. Or ignorance. Many physicians are ignorant of some aspects of the field of medicine in which they practice. They tend to think the newer pill or newer treatment must be better because it's new. Ignorance is a failure to think deeply. It is a failure to be inquisitive. It is a failure to keep an open mind.

For some patients and their families, ignorance manifests itself as unrealistic expectations. Sometimes we doctors do a lot to help patients have unrealistic expectations. Americans suffer from a massive lack of appreciation for what's realistic, given present science.

Ego, arrogance, and excessive self-confidence lead doctors to confuse what they know with what they believe. This confluence of forces leads to a closed mind and has led to advocacy of many interventions that, after years of use, were ultimately found to be not useful or even harmful.

I have met my share of doctors who would have been great snake-oil salesmen. I am amazed by the number of medical leaders who seek power and prestige through habitual lying.

Health-care providers, hospitals, drug and device manufacturers, and insurers all need to truly focus on the best interest of the patient. Some try to do the right thing, but some hospitals become more consumed with competition than with providing good care. Some drug companies seize control of medical education and advance their products through medical politics, perverse incentives, and thinly disguised (or blatant) bribery.

Take a quick inventory of everyone who benefited from the cascade of services that robbed Ralph DeAngelo of the golden years he was enjoying until that cursed health fair. The list will be long. It will begin with the manufacturers of the PSA test and go on for pages. He paid the ultimate price for becoming a one-man multiplier effect. Many health-care professionals have forgotten the definition of the word *professional*. It means a person who puts the interests of others above self-interest. This requires that one care about the welfare of others.

I hear the pundits threaten that health care is going to be rationed. I am troubled that I don't hear concern for those who need good health care and don't get it now. As I look at this mess, I realize that we don't need health-care reform. We need a health-care transformation. Americans need to change how we view health care. We need to change how it is provided and how it is consumed.

Patients and their families can be their own best advocates. They need to appreciate the scientific method and the medical literature. They need to question the source of their information and recognize that a lot of advertisements masquerade as scientific papers. They need to have skepticism and ask probing questions.

Rational health care has the potential to save millions of lives over the next several decades. It must include preventive medicine and could actually have an amazingly positive effect on the economy. To do it requires accepting that there is a significant problem, and resolving to address that problem. Patients and health-care providers must work together, constantly asking these two questions:

"What is rational?" followed by "What is reasonable?"

How do we protect ourselves, our loved ones, our neighbors? There is only one way. We do it by demanding a health-care system that can say "Prove it," a system that can say "No" and make it stick. For this to happen, real people—ideally, all 300 million of us—will have to say "Enough!"

Acknowledgments

I owe much to my mother and father, who did not just work to create opportunity for me and my sisters but made it known that they expected us to do well. My father in particular had an inherent curiosity and an intolerance of wasted opportunity. He imparted those traits in me, and the Jesuits even beyond Polo and the Reverend George R. drove it home.

I also know that it takes a village as my aunts and uncles worked hard to support the vision. I was fortunate as a number of people from the old neighborhood, from gang members to numbers runners, decided I was a good investment.

The lay teachers and sisters of the Immaculate Heart of Mary at St. Cecilia and the lay teachers and Jesuits at University of Detroit High also molded me, infusing values and warning me about the world, its dangers and its challenges, but also enticing me with its beauty. I have to mention good diocesan Basilian and Jesuit priests who befriended me and taught me.

For a time, for practical reasons of survival, I was what I will call an adjunct member of a gang in the inner city of Detroit, but I was also a member of a positive youth gang at U of D High. At "the High," as we called it, I had a group of friends with whom I debated, participated in Model United Nations, and discovered the world. I owe a lot to Michael Montgomery, Mathew Wilbert, Mark Nagel, Mark Dreyer, Tony Vizzini, and Roger Barris. They were a positive youth gang for me and are still dear friends.

I am fortunate that I have always found good influences. At the University of Chicago I was encouraged by people to whom I will always be indebted, especially Elliot Kieff, Jonathan Fanton, and John Ultmann. Later Vivian Pinn, Al Rabson, and Barry Kramer would fulfill this role.

It is fascinating, the rainbow coalition of blacks and whites and of Jews, Catholics, and Protestants.

I am of course grateful to my patients and their families and especially those who let me use their stories in this book. Patients and their experiences have been the most important element of this doctor's education.

—Otis Brawley

Notes

CHAPTER I

A history of Grady Memorial Hospital can be found in Jerry Gentry, *Grady Baby: A Year in the Life of Atlanta's Grady Hospital* (Jackson: University Press of Mississippi, 1999).

Discussion of the Grady mission with some historical perspective is found in A. G. Yancey Sr., "Medical Education in Atlanta and Health Care of Black, Minority and Low-Income People," *Journal of the National Medical Association* 80 (April 1988): 467–76.

The Tuskegee Syphilis Study and rumors about it are mentioned as reasons why African-Americans are often suspicious of medicine. The facts of the trial are frequently inaccurately conveyed even in the news media. Factual accounts have been written, such as S. M. Baker, O. W. Brawley, and L. S. Marks, "Effects of untreated syphilis in the Negro male, 1932 to 1972: A closure comes to the Tuskegee study, 2004," *Urology* 65 (2005). James H. Jones, *Bad Blood: The Tuskegee Syphilis Experiment* (1981; repr., New York: Free Press, 1993), is a history of "The Study of Untreated Syphilis in the Negro Male" (this is the official name of the Tuskegee Syphilis Study). Jones's book also mentions many of the atrocities that humans have perpetrated upon vulnerable humans and called research.

Medical Apartheid by Harriet Washington is a superb history and ethical analysis. She painstakingly researched and documented numerous medical abuses over the past two centuries, including abuses within the past decade. Many of these abuses have long been talked about in the African American oral history tradition. Washington was able to find proof of alarming truths. These findings justify distrust of the American medical profession. The literature on the fears that African-Americans have of the American medical system is portrayed in Rebecca Skloot, *The Immortal Life of Henrietta Lacks* (New York: Crown Publishers, 2010).

A number of patterns-of-care studies demonstrate that the poor as a group do not receive as high a quality of medical care as the middle class and have worse health-care outcomes: S. A. Fedewa, S. B. Edge, A. K. Stewart, M. T. Halpern, N. M. Marlow, and E. M. Ward, "Race and ethnicity are associated with delays in breast cancer treatment (2003–2006)," *Journal of Health Care for the Poor and Underserved* 22, no. 1 (2011): 128–41; A. S. Robbins, A. L. Pavluck, S. A. Fedewa, A. Y. Chen, and E. M. Ward, "Insurance status, comorbidity level, and survival among colorectal cancer patients age 18 to 64 years in the National Cancer Data Base from 2003 to 2005," *Journal of Clinical Oncology* 27, no. 22 (August 1, 2009): 3627–33 (epub, May 26, 2009); and E. Ward, H. Halpern, N. Schrag, V. Cokkinides, C. DeSantis, P. Bandi, R. Siegel, A. Stewart, and A. Jemal, "Association of insurance with cancer care utilization and outcomes," *CA: A Cancer Journal for Clinicians* 58, no. 1 (January–February 2008): 9–31 (epub, December 20, 2007).

The NCI defines the medically underserved as "individuals who lack access to primary and specialty care either because they are socioeconomically disadvantaged and they may live in areas with high poverty rates or because they reside in rural areas": http://deais.nci.nih.gov/glossary/terms ?alpha=M&currentPage=1.

Trends in breast cancer by race and ethnicity: C. Smigal, A. Jemal, E. Ward, V. Cokkinides, R. Smith, H. L. Howe, and M. Thun, "Update 2006," *CA: A Cancer Journal for Clinicians* 56, no. 3 (May–June 2006): 168–83.

A higher proportion of the African-American breast cancer population has triple negative disease compared to the population of white women with breast cancer. Triple negative breast cancer is the most serious type of breast cancer. Other forms of the disease are more aggressive, but targeted therapies can slow the progression of the disease. This is explained in L. A. Carey, E. C. Dees, L. Sawyer, et al., "The triple negative paradox: Primary tumor chemosensitivity of breast cancer subtypes," Clinical Cancer Research 13, no. 8 (April 15, 2007): 2329–34; and K. M. O'Brien,

S. R. Cole, C. K. Tse, C .M. Perou, L. A. Carey, W. D. Foulkes, L. G. Dressler, J. Geradts, and R. C. Millikan, "Intrinsic breast tumor subtypes, race, and long-term survival in the Carolina Breast Cancer Study," *Clinical Cancer Research* 16, no. 24 (December 15, 2010): 6100–6110.

U.S. breast cancer rates by race are provided by the National Cancer Institute Cancer Statistics Review at https://seer.cancer.gov.

The effect of postmenopausal hormone replacement therapy (HRT or HT) was studied in the Women's Health Initiative, a study sponsored by the National Institutes of Health.

The decline in breast cancer incidence was documented in M. Ravdin, K. A. Cronin, N. Howlader, C. D. Berg, R. T. Chlebowski, E. J. Feuer, B. K. Edwards, and D. A. Berry, "The decrease in breast cancer incidence in 2003 in the United States," *New England Journal of Medicine* 356, no. 16 (April 19, 2007); and Million Women Study Collaborators, "Patterns of use of hormone replacement therapy in one million women in Britain, 1996–2000," *BJOG* 109, no. 12 (December 2002): 1319–30.

Public law 103-43, signed in 1993 by President William Clinton, mandated the Long Island Breast Cancer Study. A good description of the study is found in M. D. Gammon, A. I. Neugut, R. M. Santella, et al., "The Long Island Breast Cancer Study Project: Description of a multi-institutional collaboration to identify environmental risk factors for breast cancer," *Breast Cancer Research and Treatment* 74, no. 3 (June 2002): 235–54.

The correlation between weight gain in childhood and earlier age of menarche is discussed in S. E. Anderson, G. E. Dallal, and A. Must, "Relative weight and race influence average age at menarche: Results from two nationally representative surveys of US girls studied 25 years apart," *Pediatrics* 111, no. 4 (pt. 1) (April 2003): 844–50.

The relation between age at menarche and race and its relationship to disease in adulthood is discussed in D. S. Freedman, L. K. Khan, M. K. Serdula, W. H. Dietz, S. R. Srinivasan, and G. S. Berenson, "Relation of age at menarche to race, time period, and anthropometric dimensions: The Bogalusa Heart Study," *Pediatrics* 110, no. 4 (October 2002): e43.

Population trends in breast cancer in Scotland can tell us a lot about breast cancer in the United States: S. B. Brown, D. J. Hole, and T. G. Cooke, "Breast cancer incidence trends in deprived and affluent Scottish women," *Breast Cancer Research and Treatment* 103, no. (June 2007):

233–38 (epub, October 11, 2006); U. Macleod, S. Ross, C. Twelves, W. D. George, C. Gillis, and G. C. Watt, "Primary and secondary care management of women with early breast cancer from affluent and deprived areas: Retrospective review of hospital and general practice records," *BMJ* 320, no. 7247 (May 27, 2000): 1442–45; C. S. Thomson, D. J. Hole, C. J. Twelves, D. H. Brewster, and R. J. Black, "Prognostic factors in women with breast cancer: Distribution by socioeconomic status and effect on differences in survival," *Journal of Epidemiology and Community Health* 55 (2001): 308–15; N. H. Gordon, "Socioeconomic factors and breast cancer in black and white Americans," *Cancer and Metastasis Reviews* 22 (2003): 55–65; B. K. Dunn, T. Agurs-Collins, D. Browne, R. Lubet, and K. A. Johnson, "Health disparities in breast cancer: Biology meets socioeconomic status," *American Journal of Public Health* 100, no. S1 (April 1, 2010): S132–39 (epub, February 10, 2010); and N. Krieger, J. T. Chen, and P. D. Waterman, "Decline in US breast cancer rates after the Women's Health Initiative: Socioeconomic and racial/ethnic differentials," *American Journal of Public Health* 100, no. 6 (June 2010): 972.

CHAPTER 2

My great-uncle Benjamin Brawley was a prolific writer. My favorites among his more than a dozen books:

The Negro Genius, first published in 1915 and last republished in 1966 by Biblo and Tannen.

Negro Builders and Heroes, first published in 1937 by the University of North Carolina Press.

A Social History of the American Negro, first published in 1923 and republished by Nabu Press in 2010.

Life expectancies of various countries come from *The World Factbook,* which is also known as the *CIA World Factbook.* This reference resource is produced by the U.S. Central Intelligence Agency with almanac-style information about the countries of the world. It is available in book form and also as a Web site, which is updated regularly: https://www.cia.gov/library/publications/the-world-factbook/.

The Organisation for Economic Co-operation and Development (OECD)
publishes data regarding more than fifty member nations. It is the best
source of health, economic, and outcomes data among countries: http://
www.oecd.org.

CHAPTER 3

Much of my concern with American medicine focuses on the tendency of
many physicians to make medical decisions without a good scientific basis:
S. Timmermans and A. Mauck, "The promises and pitfalls of evidence-
based medicine," *Health Affairs (Millwood)* 24, no. 1 (2005): 18–28; D. M.
Eddy, "Evidence-based medicine: A unified approach," *Health Affairs
(Project Hope)* 24, no. 1 (2005): 9–17, doi:10.1377/hlthaff.24.1.9. PMID
15647211; and W. A. Rogers, "Evidence-based medicine and justice:
A framework for looking at the impact of EBM upon vulnerable or
disadvantaged groups," *Journal of Medical Ethics*, 2004, retrieved December 7,
2007, http://jme.bmj.com/cgi/content/full/30/2/141. Some medical research
findings are influenced by the researchers having a financial interest in the
findings. In this study of the literature, more than one-third of research
findings have at least one author with a conflict of interest: L. S. Friedman
and E. D. Richter, "Relationship between conflicts of interest and research
results," *Journal of General Internal Medicine* 19, no. 1 (January 2004): 51–56,
doi:10.1111/j.1525-1497.2004.30617.x. PMC 1494677. PMID 14748860. Having
a conflict does not necessarily mean the researcher acted dishonestly.
The Halsted mastectomy was first performed by American surgeon William
S. Halsted of Johns Hopkins: http://www.ncbi.nlm.nih.gov/pmc/articles/
PMC1272864/?page=1.
Halsted first performed the radical mastectomy that now bears his name in
the early 1890s. He wrote about the procedure in this classic paper, whose
title is ironic because he never did a rigorous formal outcomes assessment
of the procedure: W. S. Halsted, "I. The Results of Radical Operations for
the Cure of Carcinoma of the Breast," *Annals of Surgery* 46 (1907): 1.
The modern surgical treatment of breast cancer was defined by Bernard
Fisher, Umberto Veronesi, and colleagues through a number of

well-designed clinical trials. These physicians defined how clinical
research should be done. Classic papers were B. Fisher, C. Redmond,
E. R. Fisher, et al., "Ten-year results of a randomized clinical trial
comparing radical mastectomy and total mastectomy with or without
radiation," *New England Journal of Medicine* 312, no. 11 (1985): 674; U.
Veronesi and P. Valagussa, "Inefficacy of internal mammary nodes
dissection in breast cancer surgery," *Cancer* 47 (1981): 170; U. Veronesi,
R. Saccozzi, M. Del Vecchio, et al., "Comparing radical mastectomy with
quadrantectomy, axillary dissection, and radiotherapy in patients with
small cancers of the breast," *New England Journal of Medicine* 305, no. 1
(July 2, 1981): 6–11; B. Fisher, M. Bauer, R. Margolese, et al., "Five-year
results of a randomized clinical trial comparing total mastectomy and
segmental mastectomy with or without radiation in the treatment of
breast cancer," *New England Journal of Medicine* 312, no. 11 (March 14,
1985): 665–73; B. Fisher, S. Anderson, C. K. Redmond, et al., "Reanalysis
and results after 12 years of follow-up in a randomized clinical trial
comparing total mastectomy with lumpectomy with or without
irradiation in the treatment of breast cancer," *New England Journal of
Medicine* 333 (1995): 1456; W. A. Maddox, J. T. Carpenter Jr., H. L. Laws,
et al. "A randomized prospective trial of radical (Halsted) mastectomy
versus modified radical mastectomy in 311 breast cancer patients," *Annals
of Surgery* 198 (1983): 207; B. Fisher, J. H. Jeong, S. Anderson, et al.,
"Twenty-five-year follow-up of a randomized trial comparing radical
mastectomy, total mastectomy, and total mastectomy followed by
irradiation," *New England Journal of Medicine* 347 (2002): 567; and
B. Fisher, S. Anderson, J. Bryant, et al., "Twenty-year follow-up of a
randomized trial comparing total mastectomy, lumpectomy, and
lumpectomy plus irradiation for the treatment of invasive breast cancer,"
New England Journal of Medicine 347 (2002): 1233.
A wonderful overview of breast-conserving surgery (lumpectomy) and
radiation is Early Breast Cancer Trialists' Collaborative Group, "Effects
of radiotherapy and surgery in early breast cancer. An overview of the
randomized trials," *New England Journal of Medicine* 333, no. 22 (1995):
1444.
The use of bone marrow transplant was invigorated when the following
paper was published: W. R. Bezwoda, L. Seymour, and R. D. Dansey,
"High-dose chemotherapy with hematopoietic rescue as primary

treatment for metastatic breast cancer: A randomized trial," *Journal of Clinical Oncology* 13 (1995): 2483–89.

The hope was dashed when it was revealed that other major trials did not demonstrate an advantage to the bone-marrow transplant and indeed showed a net harm. Werner Bezwoda ultimately admitted that he had falsified most of the data in his trial: D. Grady, "Breast cancer researcher admits falsifying data," *New York Times,* February 5, 2000; M. Hagmann, "Scientific misconduct. Cancer researcher sacked for alleged fraud," *Science* 287, no. 5460 (March 17, 2000): 1901–2; Philadelphia Bone Marrow Transplant Group, "Conventional-dose chemotherapy compared with high-dose chemotherapy plus autologous hematopoietic stem-cell transplantation for metastatic breast cancer," *New England Journal of Medicine* 342, no. 15 (April 13, 2000): 1069–76; M. S. Tallman, R. Gray, N. J. Robert, et al., "Conventional adjuvant chemotherapy with or without high-dose chemotherapy and autologous stem-cell transplantation in high-risk breast cancer," *New England Journal of Medicine* 349, no. 1 (July 3, 2003): 17–26; and K. H. Antman, "Overview of the six available randomized trials of high-dose chemotherapy with blood or marrow transplant in breast cancer," *Journal of the National Cancer Institute* Monograph 2001 (30): 114–16.

CHAPTER 4

Long after I began thinking of the IHM nuns as feminists because they ran things, I discovered my idea was not original, as demonstrated in the title of this book on the history of the order: *Building Sisterhood: A Feminist History of the Sisters, Servants of the Immaculate Heart of Mary,* by Sisters, Servants of the Immaculate Heart of Mary in Books.

Much has been written about the Society of Jesus. One of the books that I like is George W. Traub, S.J., *A Jesuit Education Reader* (Chicago: Loyola Press, 2008).

CHAPTER 6

An excellent overview of the history of overuse of red blood cell growth
factors can be found in F. R. Khuri, "Weighing the hazards of erythropoiesis
stimulation in patients with cancer," *New England Journal of Medicine* 356
(June 14, 2007): 2445–48.

An Amgen executive described his company's products as "white juice" and
    "red juice" during a presentation at the Goldman Sachs 28th Annual
    Global Healthcare Conference June 13, 2007.

German researcher Michael Henke discussed his surprising finding of
    harmful effects of erythropoietin in an interview with Paul Goldberg,
    "Study Tests a 'Truth' in Radiation Oncology, Raises Questions About
    Anemia Treatment," *Cancer Letter,* October 24, 2003.

Henke published his results in M. Henke, D. Mattern, M. Pepe, C. Bézay,
    C. Weissenberger, M. Werner, and F. Pajonk, "Erythropoietin receptors
    on cancer cells explain unexpected clinical findings?" *Journal of Clinical
    Oncology* 24, no. 29 (October 10, 2006): 4708–13, doi: 10.1200/
    JCO.2006.06.2737Do.

Discussion of unexpected results of a randomized trial of erythropoietin in
    breast cancer is found in Brian Leyland-Jones, on behalf of the BEST
    Investigators and Study Group, "Breast cancer trial with erythropoietin
    terminated unexpectedly," *Lancet Oncology* 4, no. 8 (August 2003): 459–60.

Henke's findings, BEST, and other studies cause many doctors to refrain
    from prescribing erythropoietin to patients with cancers of the breast and
    head and neck. Discussion in Paul Goldberg, "FDA to Once Again
    Review ESA Label to Reflect Results of Negative Studies," *Cancer Letter,*
    December 7, 2007.

The proper use of "white juice" is discussed in D. C. Dale,
    "Colony-stimulating factors for the management of neutropenia in
    cancer patients," *Drugs* 62, no. S1 (2002): S1–S15.

In mid-2010, the ACS Cancer Action Network commissioned a survey of a
nationally representative sample of the American population age eighteen and
older who say they or a member of their household has cancer or a history of
cancer: http://www.acscan.org/healthcare/cancerpoll. The study found:

  • High health costs jeopardize the ability of families affected by
    cancer to afford the care they need.

- High health costs also prevent people with cancer and their families from affording basic necessities.
- Affordability of care is a major issue for people under sixty-five.
- People with cancer and their families struggle to stay insured.

Early studies showed a benefit of 5-FU and leucovorin given adjuvantly after colon cancer surgery and removal of all known cancer for Stage III disease, and there was the suggestion of benefit for late Stage II (Stage bII) disease. Clinical trials to assess the relative efficacy of fluorouracil and leucovorin, fluorouracil and levamisole, and fluorouracil, leucovorin, and levamisole in patients with Dukes' B and C carcinoma of the colon: N. Wolmark, H. Rockette, E. Mamounas, et al., "Results from National Surgical Adjuvant Breast and Bowel Project C-04," *Journal of Clinical Oncology* 17, no. 11 (1999): 3553.

Later studies showed a benefit to using oxaliplatin in the treatment of metastatic colon cancer and later as an adjuvant therapy in surgically resected Stage III colon cancer patients: T. André, C. Boni, L. Mounedji-Boudiaf, et al., Multicenter International Study of Oxaliplatin/5-Fluorouracil/Leucovorin in the Adjuvant Treatment of Colon Cancer (MOSAIC) Investigators, "Oxaliplatin, fluorouracil, and leucovorin as adjuvant treatment for colon cancer," *New England Journal of Medicine* 350, no. 23 (2004): 2343–47; and N. Wolmark, S. Wieand, P. J. Kuebler, et al., "A phase III trial comparing FULV to FULV + oxaliplatin in stage II or III carcinoma of the colon: Survival results of NSABP Protocol C-07," *Journal of Clinical Oncology* 26 (2008): 1008.

CHAPTER 7

The controversy concerning erythropoietin (EPO, Procrit, and Aranesp) is summarized in M. R. Savona and S. M. Silver, "Erythropoietin-stimulating agents in oncology," *Cancer Journal* 14, no. 2 (March–April 2008): 75–84. Former pharmaceutical company attorneys who ran the FDA's enforcement operations blocked efforts by agency staff to stop—or at least to tone down—the Procrit ads. Internal FDA documents stemming from these unsuccessful efforts were obtained by the *Cancer Letter* and are covered in Paul Goldberg, "FDA Staff Efforts to Issue Warning Letters Were Stopped by FDA Counsel," the *Cancer Letter*, May 9, 2008.

According to a January 24, 2011, report from Bloomberg, Amgen's annual sales of Aranesp peaked at $4.1 billion in 2006 and have declined each year since after studies linked Amgen's anemia drugs to increased risk of blood clots, heart attack, and stroke, as well as tumor growth in cancer patients. Johnson & Johnson sales of erythropoietin peaked at $3.95 billion in 2003.

A twenty-eight-page summary of the reasons for higher-than-expected health-care costs in the United States: http://www.mckinsey.com/mgi/reports/pdfs/healthcare/US_healthcare_Executive_summary.pdf.

CHAPTER 8

Implantable defibrillators were developed at the University of Maryland in Baltimore in the late 1970s and early 1980s: J. A. Kastor, "Michel Mirowski and the Automatic Implantable Defibrillator," *American Journal of Cardiology* 63 (1989): 977–82, 1121–26; and J. A. Kastor, A. J. Moss, M. M. Mower, and M. L. Weisfeldt, "Michel Mirowski: A Man with a Mission," *PACE* 14 (1991): 865.

CHAPTER 9

There is a significant academic literature on the practice of medicine in the ER and especially decision-making by residents. Many patients use the ER as a place for social interaction. For the doctor, the hardest decision is when to admit. See J. M. Pines, B. R. Asplin, A. H. Kaji, R. A. Lowe, D. J. Magid, M. Raven, E. J. Weber, and D. M. Yealy, "Frequent users of emergency department services: Gaps in knowledge and a proposed research agenda," *Academic Emergency Medicine* 18, no. 6 (June 2011): e64–69, doi:10.1111/j.1553-2712.2011.01086.x; L. B. Mellick, D. van Staen, and

R. Perkin, "The role of emergency medicine in a teaching hospital: Decision making in an uncontrolled environment," *American Journal of Emergency Medicine* 11 (1993): 187; and M. C. Raven, J. C. Billings, L. R. Goldfrank, E. D. Manheimer, and M. N. Gourevitch, "Medicaid patients at high risk for frequent hospital admission: Real-time identification and remediable risks," *Journal of Urban Health* 86, no. 2 (March 2009): 230–41 (epub, December 12, 2008).

CHAPTERS 10 AND 11

For an overview of the Bakke case and the issue of affirmative action, see Howard Ball, *The Bakke Case: Race, Education, and Affirmative Action* (Lawrence: University Press of Kansas, 2000).

The acceptance of the end of life is difficult for the family and the patient: "The practice of universal presumed consent to CPR is often questioned but still in place," *American Journal of Bioethics* 10, no. 1 (January 2010): 61–67; J. P. Bishop, K. B. Brothers, J. E. Perry, and A. Ahmad, "Reviving the conversation around CPR/DNR. End of life care," *Journal of the American Medical Association* 286, no. 11 (September 19, 2001): 1349–55; and N. G. Levinsky, W. Yu, A. Ash, M. Moskowitz, G. Gazelle, O. Saynina, and E. J. Emanuel, "Influence of age on Medicare expenditures and medical care in the last year of life," *Journal of the American Medical Association* 286, no. 11 (2001): 1349–55; and A. E. Barnato, C. C. Chang, M. H. Farrell, J. R. Lave, M. S. Roberts, and D. C. Angus, "Is survival better at hospitals with higher 'end-of-life' treatment intensity?". *Medical Care* 48, no. 2 (February 2010): 125–32.

The data suggest that many doctors do not understand the limits of our abilities, and intensity of and cost of care at the end of life can vary significantly: L. R. Shugarman, S. L. Decker, and A. Bercovitz, "Demographic and social characteristics and spending at the end of life," *Journal of Pain and Symptom Management* 38, no. 1 (July 2009): 15–26.

Doctors are affected by what happens to their patients and what they do to patients. Most doctors do not discuss this. James S. Kennedy, MD, did discuss this issue in his article "Physicians' feelings about themselves and their patients," *Journal of the American Medical Association* 287 (2002): 1113–14.

CHAPTER 13

The profession of medical oncology and the National Cancer Institute were shaped by the National Cancer Act of 1971 (P.L. 92-218) signed by President Richard M. Nixon on December 23, 1971. It created many of the powers and authorities of the present-day National Cancer Institute.

CHAPTERS 14 TO 16

Informed consent was a term from the late 1950s: C. K. Daugherty, D. M. Banik, L. Janish, amd M. J. Ratain, "Quantitative analysis of ethical issues in phase I trials: A survey interview of 144 advanced cancer patients," *IRB* 22, no. 3 (May–June 2000): 6–14; and C. K. Daugherty, "Informed consent, the cancer patient, and phase I clinical trials," *Cancer Treatment and Research* 102 (2000): 77–89.

It is well established that doctors and patients put too much hope in clinical trials: K. P. Weinfurt, D. M. Seils, J. P. Tzeng, K. L. Compton, D. P. Sulmasy, A. B. Astrow, N. A. Solarino, K. A. Schulman, and N. J. Meropol, "Expectations of benefit in early-phase clinical trials: Implications for assessing the adequacy of informed consent," *Medical Decision Making* 28, no. 4 (July–August 2008): 575–81 (epub, March 31, 2008); and D. P. Sulmasy, A. B. Astrow, M. K. He, D. M. Seils, N. J. Meropol, E. Micco, and K. P. Weinfurt, "The culture of faith and hope: Patients' justifications for their high estimations of expected therapeutic benefit when enrolling in early phase oncology trials," *Cancer Journal* 116, no. 15 (August 1, 2010): 3702–11.

The "flutamide withdrawal" phenomenon (Snuffy Myers really discovered it, but he did not realize he had discovered it. He attributed the positive

response to the administration of the experimental drug suramin) was
first published in W. K. Kelly and H. I. Scher, "Prostate specific antigen
decline after antiandrogen withdrawal: The flutamide withdrawal
syndrome," *Journal of Urology* 149, no. 3 (March 1993): 607–9.
The study that showed suramin was not useful in the treatment of prostate
cancer was E. J. Small, S. Halabi, M. J. Ratain, et al., "Randomized study
of three different doses of suramin administered with a fixed dosing
schedule in patients with advanced prostate cancer: Results of intergroup
0159, cancer and leukemia group B 9480," *Journal of Clinical Oncology* 20,
no. 16 (August 15, 2002): 3369–75.
A summary of the Food and Drug Administration Oncologic Drug
Advisory Committee's review of suramin for prostate cancer was reported
in *Oncology News International* 7, no. 10 (1998).
A wonderful discussion of the early NCI is in John Laszlo, *The Cure of
Childhood Leukemia: Into the Age of Miracles* (Piscataway, NJ: Rutgers
University Press, 1996).

CHAPTER 17

The quality of surgery is extremely important in the treatment of colon
cancer: S. R. Steele, S. L. Chen, A. Stojadinovic, A. Nissan, K. Zhu, G. E.
Peoples, and A. Bilchik, "The impact of age on quality measure adherence
in colon cancer," *Journal of the American College of Surgeons* 213, no. 1
(July 2011): 95–103; discussion, 104–5 (epub, May 20, 2011).
A good review of what is known, what is not known, and what is believed
regarding chemotherapy after surgical removal of all known colon cancer
is H. C. Moore and D. G. Haller, "Adjuvant therapy of colon cancer,"
Seminars in Oncology 26, no. 5 (1999): 545.
The trial looking specifically at Stage II disease (keep in mind that the
patient had an even better prognosis Stage I): W. Schippinger,
H. Samonigg, R. Schaberl-Moser, et al., Austrian Breast and Colorectal
Cancer Study Group, "A prospective randomised phase III trial of adjuvant
chemotherapy with 5-fluorouracil and leucovorin in patients with stage II
colon cancer," *British Journal of Cancer* 97, no. 8 (2007): 1021.

A review of leukemias and blood diseases caused by cancer chemotherapy is
in L. A. Godley and R. A. Larson, "Therapy-related myeloid leukemia,"
Seminars in Oncology 35 (2008): 418.

Colon cancer chemotherapy poses significant neurological and other
quality-of-life issues, as discussed in I. Chau, A. R. Norman, D.
Cunningham, et al., "Longitudinal quality of life and quality adjusted
survival in a randomised controlled trial comparing six months of bolus
fluorouracil/leucovorin vs. twelve weeks of protracted venous infusion
fluorouracil as adjuvant chemotherapy for colorectal cancer," *European
Journal of Cancer* 41, no. 11 (2005): 1551; and S. R. Land, J. A. Kopec,
R. S. Cecchini, et al., "Neurotoxicity from oxaliplatin combined with
weekly bolus fluorouracil and leucovorin as surgical adjuvant
chemotherapy for stage II and III colon cancer: NSABP C-07," *Journal
of Clinical Oncology* 25, no. 16 (2007): 2205.

CHAPTER 18

Gonadotropin-releasing hormone (GnRH) agonists such as leuprolide and
Zoladex are used in the treatment of metastatic prostate cancer. The
American Society of Clinical Oncology has established guidelines to define
their appropriate use: D. A. Loblaw, K. S. Virgo, R. Nam, et al., "Initial
hormonal management of androgen-sensitive metastatic, recurrent, or
progressive prostate cancer: 2006 update of an American Society of Clinical
Oncology practice guideline," *Journal of Clinical Oncology* 25 (2007): 1596.

In a well-done study, the high reimbursement for androgen deprivation
therapy seems to be correlated with overuse and misuse of the drugs.
Lowering physician reimbursement seemed to be correlated with less
misuse of these drugs: V. B. Shahinian, Y. F. Kuo, and S. M. Gilbert,
"Reimbursement policy and androgen-deprivation therapy for prostate
cancer," *New England Journal of Medicine* 363, no. 19 (November 4, 2010):
1822–32.

This is a classic paper on the use of diethylstilbestrol in prostate cancer: D. P.
Byar and D. K. Corle, "Hormone therapy for prostate cancer: Results of

the Veterans Administration Cooperative Urological Research Group studies," NCI Monograph, 1988; and D. P. Byar, "Proceedings: The Veterans Administration Cooperative Urological Research Group's studies of cancer of the prostate," *Cancer Journal* 32, no. 5 (1973): 1126.
Prilosec sales reached their peak globally in 2000, reaching $6.1 billion, accounting for 35 percent of all product sales in this drug class: http:// www.panopharma.com/world_pharma_sales_2000.htm. Sales remained constant in 2001: http://www.panopharma.com/world_pharma_sales _2001.htm. By 2002, Prilosec sales dropped to $5.2 billion worldwide, as a result of competition and AstraZeneca's promotion of its follow-up product, Nexium (esomeprazole): http://www.panopharma.com/ world_pharma_sales_2002.htm. By 2005, both Prilosec and omeprazole were among the top-one-hundred-selling drugs in the United States, with AstraZeneca's follow-on isomeric replacement, Nexium, in the top thirty: http://www.rxlist.com/script/main /art.asp?articlekey=79509. By 2007, Nexium was the second-largest-selling drug in the United States, with sales of $4.355 billion; prescription Prilosec still accounted for another $174 million in sales (the 171st-largest-selling product): http://www.drugs .com/top200.html. By 2007, generic omeprazole was the twenty-fourth-most-prescribed drug in the United States, and the tenth-largest-selling generic pharmaceutical product, with sales of more than $835 million, a 30 percent increase over 2006: http://drugtopics.modernmedicine.com/ drugtopics/data/articlestandard//drugtopics/ 072008/491181/ article.pdf; and http://drugtopics.modernmedicine.com/drugtopics/data/article standard//drugtopics /102008/500218/article.pdf.
The development of Nexium as a successor to Prilosec was reported on by Malcolm Gladwell, "High Prices: How to Think about Prescription Drugs," *New Yorker,* October 25, 2004. The trials that made us appreciate that most nonsteroidal anti-inflammatory drugs and especially rofecoxib (Vioxx) and celecoxib (Celebrex) increased risk of heart attack and stroke were J. A. Baron, R. S. Sandler, R. S. Bresalier, et al., APPROVe Trial Investigators, "A randomized trial of rofecoxib for the chemoprevention of colorectal adenomas," *Gastroenterology* 131, no. 6 (December 2006): 1674–82; and S. D. Solomon, J. J. V. McMurray, M. A. Pfeffer, et al., for the Adenoma Prevention with Celecoxib (APC) Study Investigators, "Cardiovascular risk associated with celecoxib in a clinical trial for

colorectal adenoma prevention," *New England Journal of Medicine* 352 (2005): 1071–80.

Estimated risk of radiation-induced cancer due to medical radiation varies. Some estimate that that 1 percent of all cancers in the United States are due to diagnostic radiation: J. Hall and D. J. Brenner, "Cancer risks after radiation exposure in middle age," *Journal of the National Cancer Institute* 102, no. 21 (2010): 1628; and A. J. Einstein, M. J. Henzlova, and S. Rajagopalan, "Estimating risk of cancer associated with radiation exposure from 64-slice computed tomography coronary angiography," Journal of the American Medical Association 298, no. 3 (2007): 317.

Despite its popularity, robotic surgery has not been proven superior to conventional surgery in the surgeries for which it is most commonly used: A. Mottrie, G. De Naeyer, G. Novara, and V. Ficarra, "Robotic radical prostatectomy: A critical analysis of the impact on cancer control," *Current Opinion in Urology* 21, no. 3 (May 2011): 179–84; and M. A. Orvieto, G. J. Decastro, Q. D. Trinh, C. Jeldres, M. H. Katz, V. R. Patel, and K. C. Zorn, "Oncological and functional outcomes after robot-assisted radical cystectomy: Critical review of current status," *Urology,* September 2, 2011.

A discussion of the limited scientific data to support for the use of IMRT: M. T. Guerrero Urbano and C. M. Nutting, "Clinical use of intensity-modulated radiotherapy: Part II," *British Journal of Radiology* 77, no. 915 (2004): 177.

CHAPTER 21

The prostate portion of the Prostate, Lung, Colorectol and Ovarian (PLCO) Screening Trial was published in G. L. Andriole, E. D. Crawford, R. L. Grubb 3rd, et al., "Mortality results from a randomized prostate-cancer screening trial," *New England Journal of Medicine* 360 (2009): 1310.

The European study is F. H. Schröder, J. Hugosson, M. J. Roobol, et al., "Screening and prostate-cancer mortality in a randomized European study," *New England Journal of Medicine* 360 (2009): 1320.

Other important prostate cancer studies include I. M. Thompson,
D. K. Pauler, P. J. Goodman, et. al., "Prevalence of prostate cancer
among men with a prostate-specific antigen level < or = 4.0 ng per
milliliter," *New England Journal of Medicine* 350, no. 22 (May 27, 2004):
2239–46, erratum in *New England Journal of Medicine* 351, no. 14
(September 30, 2004): 1470; and I. M. Thompson, P. J. Goodman,
C. M. Tangen, et al., "The influence of finasteride on the development
of prostate cancer," *New England Journal of Medicine* 349, no. 3
(July 17, 2003): 215–24.

CHAPTER 22

The American Urological Association prostate cancer best-practice statement
can be found at http://www.auanet.org/content/media/psa09.pdf.
The lung cancer screening trial: National Lung Screening Trial
    Research Team, D. R. Aberle, A. M. Adams, C. D. Berg, et al.,
    "Reduced lung-cancer mortality with low-dose computed tomographic
    screening," *New England Journal of Medicine* 365, no. 5 (August 4,
    2011): 395–409.
The study of the process used to prepare 431 guidelines: R. Grilli,
    N. Magrini, A. Penna, G. Mura, and A. Liberati, "Practice guidelines
    developed by specialty societies: The need for a critical appraisal," *Lancet*
    355, no. 9198 (January 8, 2000): 103–6.

CHAPTER 23

David Ransohoff's fellowship paper is D. F. Ransohoff and A. R. Feinstein,
"Problems of spectrum and bias in evaluating the efficacy of diagnostic
tests," *New England Journal of Medicine* 299, no. 17 (October 26, 1978):
926–30.

CHAPTER 24

The history of breast cancer advocacy and Project LEAD is based on interviews with Fran Visco, Kay Dickersin, and Susan Love. One excellent account appears in *Dr. Susan Love's Breast Book*, 5th ed. (New York: Da Capo, a Merloyd Lawrence Book, 2010).